Men's Health

Dedication:
To all the boys and men whose lives have motivated us
to write this book

Men's Health
Perspectives, Diversity and Paradox

Mike Luck
Margaret Bamford

and

Peter Williamson

Blackwell Science

© 2000 by
Blackwell Science Ltd
Editorial Offices:
Osney Mead, Oxford OX2 0EL
25 John Street, London WC1N 2BL
23 Ainslie Place, Edinburgh EH3 6AJ
350 Main Street, Malden
  MA 02148 5018, USA
54 University Street, Carlton
  Victoria 3053, Australia
10, rue Casimir Delavigne
  75006 Paris, France

Other Editorial Offices:

Blackwell Wissenschafts-Verlag GmbH
Kurfürstendamm 57
10707 Berlin, Germany

Blackwell Science KK
MG Kodenmacho Building
7–10 Kodenmacho Nihombashi
Chuo-ku, Tokyo 104, Japan

This Edition published 2000

Set in 10/12pt Times
by DP Photosetting, Aylesbury, Bucks

DISTRIBUTORS

Marston Book Services Ltd
PO Box 269
Abingdon
Oxon OX14 4YN
(*Orders:* Tel: 01235 465500
              Fax: 01235 465555)

USA
Blackwell Science, Inc.
Commerce Place
350 Main Street
Malden, MA 02148 5018
(*Orders:* Tel: 800 759 6102
              781 388 8250
              Fax: 781 388 8255)

Canada
Login Brothers Book Company
324 Saulteaux Crescent
Winnipeg, Manitoba R3J 3T2
(*Orders:* Tel: 204 837-2987
              Fax: 204 837-3116)

Australia
Blackwell Science Pty Ltd
54 University Street
Carlton, Victoria 3053
(*Orders:* Tel: 03 9347 0300
              Fax: 03 9347 5001)

A catalogue record for this title is available
from the British Library

ISBN 0-632-05288-0

Library of Congress
Cataloging-in-Publication Data
Luck, Mike.
    Men's health: perspectives, diversity,
and paradox/by Mike Luck, Margaret
Bamford, and Peter Williamson.
        p.   cm.
    Includes bibliographical references and
index.   [ADJUST 008?]
    ISBN 978-0-632-05288-2
    1. Men—Health and hygiene.
I. Bamford, Margaret.   II. Williamson,
Peter.   III. Title.
    [DNLM: 1. Health.   2. Men.
    WA 300 L941m 1999]
RA777.8.L83   1999
613'.04234—dc21
DNLM/DLC
for Library of Congress   99-32983
                                              CIP

For further information on
Blackwell Science, visit our website:
www.blackwell-science.com

Contents

List of Figures

Icons Used in this Text

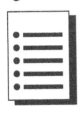   *Personal Stories*

   Exhortations

   Major Summary Points

List of Tables

List of Personal Stories

Acknowledgements

Mike Luck

My motivation, experience and writing have been encouraged by many people whom I have tried to acknowledge below.

In 1991 five men, Peter Bruckenwell, David Jackson, Jim Wallace, Jonk Watts and myself met to discuss how to start a project on men's health. Our discussion led to the writings which were published by Community Health UK under the title *The Crisis in Men's Health* (Bruckenwell *et al.* 1995). The positive responses to this publication encouraged me to continue to explore the topic.

David Jackson has continued to be a good friend and constructive critic throughout this project.

A Men's Health Network was set up in South Warwickshire in 1994 with the main purpose of bringing together men and women who are working on men's health issues. The network has continued to provide a focus for ideas and support. The following people have provided many useful comments and detailed suggestions and support: Liz Biolik, the late Richard de Groot, Dhillon, Phil Jenkins, Chris Jones, Mrs Kohli, Terry Leather, Dick Leith, Ian Lucas, Felix Lunt, Bill Ollis, Tanis Ratcliffe, Guy Shennan, Steve Smith, Lillian Somervaille, Alan Taman, John Taylor, Simon Warren, Patrick Wilson, Chris Wood.

Penny Broad has continued with great skill and enthusiasm to promote men's health on the agenda of the Warwickshire Health Authority and has provided me with information and support.

Thanks to Jane Winder for the figures and tables, Debbie Evans for Figure 9.1, and Jean Elkington for IT support especially with the e-mail files.

Thanks to Ann for lots of support especially when I had the 'flu.

Peter Williamson

Janet Baker, Assistant Director of Public Health, NHSE-West Midlands; Dr. Steve Bridgeman, Consultant in Public Health Medicine, North

Staffordshire Health Authority; Penny Broad, Health Promotion Specialist, South Warwickshire Health Promotion Service; Lee Cook, Sexual Health Worker and Lois Swift, Associate Director of Public Health, Sandwell Health Authority; Phil Deakin, Health Promotion Specialist, Coventry Health Authority; Neil Field, Drug Action Team Co-ordinator, Solihull Health Authority; Meryl Johnson, Health Promotion Co-ordinator, Worcestershire Health Authority; Brian Mackenzie, Head of Health-Works, Dorset; Julian Reeves, Deputy Director of Health Promotion, Herefordshire Health Authority; Dr Neil Stevenson, GP, Norfolk; and Jon Topham, Health Promotion Manager, South Staffordshire Health Authority.

Rob Lloyd-Owen, MEN-D, Feisal Jassat, Kirklees Metropolitan Council, and Professor Chris Worth, Calderdale and Kirklees Health Authority, for their information on the Kirklees Men's Health Network.

Andrew Gow, Policy Analyst, Health Services Policy Branch, New South Wales Health Department, Australia; Dr. Ulrich J. Grueninger, Head of the Health Strategy Development Unit, Department of Public Health, Swiss Federal Office of Public Health, Koeniz, Berne, Switzerland; Michael Kakakios, Policy Manager, Health Services Policy Branch, New South Wales Health Department, Australia; Julia Muschner, Project Co-ordinator, Gesundes Dresden, Germany; David Simpson, Health Promotion Specialist, North Western Health Board, Republic of Ireland; Dr. Hannes Schmidl, Department of Health Planning, Vienna, and Professor Anita Schmeiser-Rieder, University of Vienna, Austria; Stephen Rue, Policy Officer, Tasmanian Department of Community and Health Services.

Professor Hilary Graham, Economic and Social Research Council, University of Lancaster; Geoff Latham, Health Strategy Unit, and Dr. Sanjai Gupta and Joe Monks, Health Promotion Division, Department of Health; Maggie Robinson, Community Education Development Centre, Coventry; Debbie Matthews, Project Officer Healthy Sheffield; Dr Paul Aveyard, Senior Registrar in Public Health, Birmingham Health Authority; Peter Lumb, Department of Social Work and Social Policy, University of South Australia, Adelaide; the secretariat of World Health Organization's Health For All programme, Geneva, Switzerland.

David Jackson and Chris Bristow, Nottingham Men's Health Forum; Terry Leather, South Warwickshire Men's Health Network.

The authors would like to thank the following copyright holders for permission to reproduce Figures and Tables: Ashgate Publishing Limited, Figure 4.7; Professor Muriel Blaxter, Figure 4.8, Figure 4.9; Professor Joan Busfield, Figure 4.1; Elsevier Science Ltd, Figure 2.9, Figure 2.10; Professor Anne Johnson, Figure 4.5, Figure 4.6; Professor Janice Morse, Figure 4.10; NHS Executive West Midlands, Figure 4.3, Figure 4.4; Office for National

Statistics, Table 2.2, Figure 2.2, Figure 2.3, Figure 2.4, Figure 2.8; Office of Population Censuses and Surveys, Table 2.1, Figure 2.1, Figure 2.6; Policy Studies Institute, Table 2.3, Table 2.4, Table 4.3, Table 4.4, Table 4.5, Table 4.6, Table 4.7, Table 4.8, Figure 4.2; David Sallah, Table 4.1, Table 4.2; Dr Kaye Wellings, Table 3.1, Table 4.9, Figure 3.1; Margaret Whitehead, Figure 9.2; Professor Richard Wilkinson, Figure 2.5.

Thanks to the anonymous reviewers and to Jan Rose for comments and suggestions.

Foreword

'Health is ... profoundly unequal. Health inequality runs throughout life ... it exists between men and women...'

This statement from the White Paper *Saving Lives – Our Healthier Nation*[1] confirms the vital work still necessary to promote men's health issues. This is not only important to boys and men themselves but to decision makers from a wide range of statutory and non-statutory agencies and ultimately government itself.

The publication of the Chief Medical Officer's 1992 Annual Report[2] was one of the first reports to detail men's health issues nationally. Since then a relatively small number of other theses, reports and books have been issued to continue to raise awareness and suggestions on tackling effectively men's health issues. Indeed, the message and intentions were expressed simply but profoundly in the words of one colleague in 1994 (Professor Rod Griffiths, West Midlands Regional Director of Public Health) '... the most important new conclusion that I have now reached is that something should be done about the health of men...'[3]

In recent years, the outcomes of a heightened social awareness of issues of equal opportunities have led to policy makers giving increased attention to women's health. In fact, the most recent Expert Report (*The Acheson Report*) on Inequalities in Health[4] has highlighted the health of mothers and families for particular action.

The profound inequalities in men's and boy's health, however, are becoming increasingly well known. *Our Healthier Nation* highlights the wide health gap already existing in each of the main disease groups. The fact that life expectancy at birth currently for a boy is about five years less than for a girl born at the same time must surely be disturbing.

Some positive progress on reducing the impact to male health for specific cancers (e.g. prostate and testicular) can be reported and is discussed in this important book. However, concentrating on these areas ignores the important effects of psycho-social pressures on men within modern society. Indeed, we can argue that men, in so far as they continue to hold positions of power and influence in many areas of social life, perhaps contribute to the incidence of ill health not only among themselves but also among women (and children).

It is clear that men's health is shaped by many social influences. Cultural images of manhood may cause younger males to indulge in risk-taking behaviour; societal influences in recent years have included less uses of men for labour; and high male unemployment rates contribute to mental ill-health.

However, on a positive note, we have seen much greater promotional efforts nationally to raise men's health issues through, for example, the use of magazines and the wider media. Some local men's health networks have developed with varying degrees of success. To date, there have been relatively few attempts to provide an overview of men's health. This book, however, does just that in providing local to international perspectives. The interested reader, male or female, policy-maker or single parent, will find some fascinating material to ponder and act on. Given current local, national and international policy to reduce inequalities in health, this book should be seen as a landmark for all involved in promoting and trying to improve male health.

Professor Chris Worth
Executive Director of Public Health
Calderdale and Kirklees Health Authority
Huddersfield, UK

References

1. Secretary of State for Health. *Saving Lives – Our Healthier Nation*. CM 4386. London: The Stationery Office, 1999.

2. Chief Medical Officer. *On the State of The Public Health for the Year 1992*. London: HMSO, 1993.

3. Griffiths, R. *Call for Action on Men's Health*. Annual Report of the West Midlands Regional Director of Public Health. Birmingham: West Midlands RHA, 1994.

4. Independent Inquiry into Inequalities in Health. Report of the Independent Inquiry into Inequalities in Health. London: The Stationery Office, 1999. Chairman: Sir Donald Acheson.

Chapter 1

Is There a Crisis in Men's Health?

In this chapter we:

- debate the proposition that there is a crisis in men's health;
- explain the purpose of the book and provide an outline to help readers with different needs to extract the maximum benefit from the book;
- compare the recent emergence of interest in men's health with the well established women's health movement;
- recommend that readers should relate their personal knowledge and experience of a man's health to the wider social and political analysis.

Introduction

> **Box 1.1: Men on their health**
>
> 'People who go to the doctor are all women and children ... and people who are really ill.'
>
> 'I don't go to the doctor because it can't be all that serious and I'm just too busy.'
>
> 'The wife said I had to come ... [reported to GP].'
>
> 'I would have been back at work sooner but the wife said I hadn't eaten for 24 hours and so shouldn't be driving.'
>
> Source: Bruckenwell *et al.*, 1995, pp. 3–4.

In this chapter our aim is to explain to the reader our purpose in writing the book and to explain our approach and provide an outline of the contents so that the reader can gain maximum benefit relative to his or her knowledge and experience.

This book has emerged from several years experience of men talking to each other about their own health attitudes and behaviour. More recently men and women have been trying to generalise these individual experiences and relate them to the gender socialisation process, and to seek policies and practices which will improve boys' and men's health. We hope that each reader, male and female, can retain this balance between the personal and political.

We have been strongly influenced by the much longer tradition of action, research and writing about women's health. Nevertheless, the men and women who are involved in men's health should not try to replicate directly the experience of the women's health movement. One important difference, for example, is that we have a much smaller research base on men's health from a gender perspective and far fewer personal stories by men.

Despite the restrictions outlined in the paragraph above, we have been surprised to find as the writing of this book began that we had much more material than we could fit into one book. We have, therefore, decided to put the main emphasis on the health of men in the 'working years', from 16 to 59 years old approximately. It is, of course, impossible to draw arbitrary age lines and it has been necessary to include a good deal of material about infants and boys because the socialisation in these early years has such a profound influence throughout life.

The 'crisis'

There is a growing interest in the subject of men's health and it has even been described as a 'crisis' (Bruckenwell *et al.*, 1995). What grounds are there for these views? Much of the interest, or alarm, has arisen from comparisons of men's and women's mortality and morbidity. Examples from the Chief Medical Officer's 1992 Annual Report (DOH, 1993) are:

- *Life expectancy*: males die on average five years younger than females in the 1990s. However, while life expectancy has increased during this century, the difference between males and females has not changed significantly (p. 80).
- *Mortality by age*: the male death rate is higher than the female death rate in all age groups. The greatest excess is in young adults due mainly to accidents, suicide and AIDS. Deaths in this age group have been increasing (p. 81).
- *International comparisons*: When life expectancy at birth for females and males is compared between 16 industrialised countries the UK comes somewhere in the middle (p. 82).

What these indicators suggest is that although there have not been any sudden changes in the statistics for mortality and life expectancy, with the exception of deaths of young adults, more detailed attention is being given to data that were already available. This increase in attention comes both from within the NHS and from broader social trends.

Within the NHS, the development of the national health strategy *The Health Of The Nation* (DOH, 1992), based on the selection of five key areas with numerical targets, has led to the more detailed scrutiny of health statistics at national and district levels. The recent report *Variations In Health* (DOH, 1996a) examines differences in health between population groups and suggests that there is plenty of scope for improvement. The health of males offers such an opportunity.

There are social trends which have been giving publicity to controversies about boys and men such as underachievement in education, teenage crime and joyriding. Men's health needs to be related to these broader trends. In schools, attention is being given to 'boys' underachievement' (Jackson, 1996).

> The old incentives, for many boys, to become respectable, working men – with status, pride, security – are now breaking apart ... (p. 3)
> And that often means buying into a culture of aggressive, heterosexual manliness that deliberately rejects school learning as an unmanly activity. (p. 13)

It seems likely that aggressive, heterosexual manliness may be linked to rejection of healthy behaviours. The high rate of long-term unemployment is seen to affect men since work has been such a significant part of the male identity and may be a contributor to the increase in young men's suicides. Among the socio-demographic factors associated with increased risk of suicide are:

- male;
- divorced, widowed, single;
- unemployed or retired;
- living alone (socially isolated) (HAS, 1995, p. 10).

Male violence at all ages from childhood into adulthood is being debated. Connell (1995) describes the routine violence in the lives of young blue-collar men in Australia:

> The interviews mention bullying and outrageous canings at school, assaulting a teacher, fights with siblings and parents, brawls in playgrounds and at parties, being arrested, assaults in reform school and gaol, bashings of women and gay men, individual fist fights and pulling a knife (Connell, 1995, p. 98)

There is political and academic debate about men in relationships, 'the family' and in parenting (Luczynski, 1996; Lloyd and Wood, 1996).

Thus, although the 'objective facts' about masculinity and men's health have not changed dramatically, the attention given has definitely increased. There are, of course, advantages and disadvantages to this development. The danger is that the political spotlight will lead to expectations of quick solutions and, if these are not forthcoming, there will be a sudden loss of interest and the topic of men's health will recede into the shadows. We shall argue that quick solutions are unlikely and, therefore, those of us who want to see men's health improve have to look for a strategy of long-term development. Nevertheless, we hope to provide enough opportunities for short-term progress to keep men's health on the agenda.

The purpose of the book

The purpose of this book is to examine and clarify what is known about the socialisation of boys and men and how this affects the way in which they maintain their health, how they respond to illness and how they do or do not seek help. We then use this understanding as a basis for exploring how national, regional and local strategies can be developed to improve boys' and men's health.

Personal perspectives

When a group of men (including one of the authors, Mike Luck) met in 1991 to discuss men's health, we soon realised that we had only a limited knowledge of the statistics which showed that men die younger than women on average. We were also aware of anecdotal evidence that men are reluctant to recognise and act on their health needs. We decided to start by looking at our personal experiences of health and illness. Eventually we wrote some of this down and it has been published as *The Crisis in Men's Health* (Bruckenwell *et al.*, 1995).

Box 1.2: Mike

Today I woke up about 5 a.m. with a sense of a threatening dream, but I could not remember it in any detail. I needed to pee. That feels like a signal of getting older, that my bladder is more insistent and short-term. I am vaguely aware that I should find out about the prostate, many men have this operation, it can affect sexual performance, but I keep putting off finding out. Most of the men I know well are quite a bit younger so they won't want to discuss peeing, bladder control and the prostate ...

I make a cup of tea ... I take the mug back to my room and get ready to start my exercises. These exercises are a crucial event in my day ... my body definitely needs these movements in order to identify its parts and make its connections. If I am feeling bad at the start I can usually persuade myself to do the first one only, then I can just find the purpose to move on to the second and so on. So usually I do get through a whole sequence, about 25 minutes.

Source: Bruckenwell *et al.*, 1995, pp. 40–41.

There are, of course, many women involved with boys' and men's health including mothers, partners, carers and health staff. Their views are important.

Box 1.3: Margaret

I am interested in men's health at three levels: the personal consequences for the individual; the effects of men in a family not having optimum health; and the consequences of men's ill health on their community. I am particularly interested in the adverse effects of work on men's health.

When I was about eleven, my father got a job as undermanager in a pit on the coast in Cumberland. The pit took its coal from under the seabed, they mined under the sea. In a local village that year about 40 families of women and children were going to Yugoslavia as guests of the Yugoslavian Miners' Association for a holiday. Every one of those families had lost a male member at work in the local mine. The sea had come into the mine workings and drowned a whole shift of men. I remember being appalled that someone could go to work and then be killed.

Having lived in mining communities for most of my formative years I had other experiences of work killing men. Sometimes this was as a result of accident or injury, sometimes by disease. My own father died of coal miner's pneumoconiosis, coal dust on the lungs, a slow and distressing way to die.

I also had more direct experience of work killing men when I worked as a colliery nursing officer in the South Yorkshire coalfields in the late 1960s. Because of my job, I was usually the one who together with a local policeman would visit the family with the bad news.

So, I have an abiding interest in men's health, particularly those areas of work where interventions can prevent ill health. The workplace with all its changes is still a good place to encourage good health behaviours, promote health and prevent ill health.

We would like the reader, male or female, to take the time to consider their own involvement with boys' and men's health from the personal perspective as well as the professional perspective. Box 1.4 suggests an exercise which can be carried out individually and also which we have used in workshops in order to sensitise participants to the importance of reflecting on their own experience.

To make further progress, it seemed necessary to move on from the personal experiences of five men and to collect and organise information on a much wider scale, which is the purpose of this book. But we consider that it is important to maintain both the personal and political perspectives throughout. We have to ensure that the messages reach individual men in their own contexts and with their personal histories. Examples of the issues

> **Box 1.4: Reader's experience of a man's health**
>
> For 60 seconds close your eyes and:
>
> *for a man* – think of an event connected with your health and concentrate on the feelings, emotions, that this brought up for you at the time;
>
> *for a woman* – think of a health event for a man you know well such as father, brother, son, partner or close friend and try to imagine the feelings, emotions, that this brought up for the man (if that is difficult think about an event connected with your own health).
>
> In a workshop, it may be useful to do this exercise in pairs, telling your partner about your event and the feelings and then listening to your partner's story.

which have emerged from personal perspectives show that some of the common attitudes of men towards their own health are:

- seeking help is unmanly;
- maintaining 'the stiff upper lip';
- depending on women to manage men's health.

Men's health

The evolution of interest in men's health has come much later than that in women's health outlined in the next section. In contrast with the grass roots development of women's health within a much wider political feminist consciousness, men's health has been a mixture of small local initiatives and top-down professional development with, as yet, quite a small lobby. It might easily fade away and be supplanted by other issues because it is not embedded within a wider political men's movement.

The first official recognition that men's health was on the political agenda came in the 1992 Annual Report of the Chief Medical Officer for England and Wales (DOH, 1993). This contained an extensive review of mortality and morbidity data and what is known of health-related behaviour. It ended with a short section 'Improving the health of men' which acknowledged that there was limited evidence on causes and effective interventions:

> Gender differences in mortality and morbidity undoubtedly exist: but what are they caused by and what can be done about them? There is increasing evidence that many of the patterns observed stem from differences in health-related behaviour, which may be influenced by the knowledge, attitudes and beliefs of men. (DOH, 1993, p.105)

The first national Men's Health Conference was held on 16 September 1994, organised by the East Midlands Men's Health Network. There were 170 participants from a wide range of statutory and voluntary agencies, including occupational health, community development, health promotion, prison health, and practice nurses and HIV/AIDS workers. The keynote speakers were: Dr Diana McInnes, a Principal Medical Officer at the Department of Health, who explained how men's health fits into the Health of the Nation strategy (although prostate and testicular cancer do not have specific targets); Trefor Lloyd, of Working With Men, talked about 'Promoting men's health' based on his series of consultancies for the Health Education Authority; Dr Sian Griffiths, the Director of Public Health for Oxfordshire Health Authority, described their approach to purchasing services for men's health in the context of the five year health strategy. In the morning, workshops were held with the aim of sharing experiences and interests, particularly between different agencies. In the afternoon, workshops were held covering a wide range of topics including: men, unemployment and health; testicular self-examination; the health needs of black men. Two important documents had been prepared for the conference: 'The men's health factsheet' which provided an excellent summary of mortality data, risk factors, social factors, and trends; and 'Purchasing health services for men'.

The second national Men's Health Conference was held on 15 December 1995. The two keynote speakers were David Morgan, who spoke about the links between gender and health, and Vic Seidler, who spoke about how aspiring to be masculine can lead to ill health. Both these speakers are sociologists and provided a contrast to the three keynote speakers at the first national conference who were either employed in or consultants to the NHS. The format of the workshops was similar to those at the first national conference: sharing and networking in the morning, followed by a wide selection of theme workshops in the afternoon.

These two national Men's Health Conferences have shown that there was a considerable degree of interest by health and other professionals and voluntary workers in the subject. It had been valuable to meet and share ideas and experiences. But, in order to make concrete progress, steps were needed to develop a sound research base, to share information and resources on a regular basis, and to involve health authorities and GP fundholders (now absorbed into Primary Care Groups) as commissioners of health.

The next step was the setting up of the National Men's Health Resource Centre by the East Midlands Men's Health Network. The Network's catalogue (now in 2nd edition, 1997) lists 183 resources including books, training packs, groupwork games, videos, posters and leaflets. The headings used to catalogue the resources are shown below:

- abuse;
- attitudes;
- bibliography;
- cancer;
- children;
- general health;
- learning difficulties;
- media;
- mental health;
- mortality;
- offenders;
- parenting;
- probation;
- rape;
- reports;
- sex education;
- sexual health;
- social work.

This list provides a useful framework for thinking about men's health in the widest context.

A number of local men's health networks have been set up including the East Midlands, Sheffield, Leicester, Chorley and South Ribble, Nottingham, Liverpool, North Derbyshire, South Warwickshire and Kirklees. These have provided useful opportunities for local networking, developing knowledge, and some local lobbying of NHS health authorities and trusts. The Kirklees Men's Health Network has carried out a research project; the Nottingham Men's Health Forum is currently developing a programme for training staff in gender awareness; the Warwickshire Men's Health Network intends to produce a leaflet for purchasers of health care.

Publications on men's health are beginning to emerge. There are now four popular manuals. Banks (1997) has produced a guide to 20 topics which is entertaining and accessible with personal anecdotes and cartoons. Brewer (1995) has written a detailed reference book 360 pages long. Part I contains ten chapters on sexual health; Part II has six chapters on illness and disease; and Part III is concerned with nutrition and lifestyle. Bradford's (1995) book is similar in approach to Brewer and is even longer at 490 pages. It is organised into 19 chapters ranging from 'Acne' to 'Complementary medicine', providing detailed information including resources and further contact addresses. Carroll's (1994) book is organised around health themes, rather than illness which is the main focus of the other three books. The chapters include 'How to stay physically healthy' and 'Coping with stress', and there is a chapter on 'Fatherhood'.

Women's health

We can learn a lot by examining how women's health has developed as a political and professional issue over the last 20 years. There are lessons we can adopt for men's health but there are very significant differences which should not be ignored. Women's health has largely developed from the grass roots: women got together and decided that they wanted to take control from the medical profession or at least share it with them more equally. Health emerged as an issue from a much wider feminist agenda in the 1970s. The first major text *Our Bodies Ourselves* was published in the USA (Boston Women's Health Collective, 1973), and the first British edition was published five years later.

> The history of this book ... began in a small discussion group... We had all experienced frustration and anger towards specific doctors and the medical maze in general... As we talked we began to realize how little we knew about our own bodies... The results of our findings were used to present courses for other women... *We feel that it would be best for men to do what we have done for themselves.* [emphasis added] (Phillips and Rakusen, revised 1996, p. 11)

Since that time, in addition to women individually and collectively exerting more control over their bodies and the delivery of health services, there has been an extensive development of academic research and publication about women's health (for example Oakley 1981, Graham 1993, Doyal 1995). Doyal's book is particularly valuable because she puts women's health in an international perspective and she attempts to avoid the traps of 'crude universalism' and of 'crude difference theories'. She has a relevant message about men's health:

> This is not a book about the health of both sexes. It is quite unapologetically a book about women ... it would be one measure of the book's success if the framework presented here were adapted for *a similar study of the influence of gender divisions on men's health.* [emphasis added] (Doyal, 1995, p. 3)

Concepts of health

What is meant by 'health' has concentrated people's minds for some considerable time. There are some widely agreed international definitions:

> The extent to which an individual or group is able, on the one hand, to realise aspirations and satisfy needs and on the other hand, to change or cope with the environment. Health is therefore seen as a resource for everyday life, not the objective of living: it is a positive concept emphasizing social and personal resources as well as physical capacities. (WHO, 1985, p. 36)

It is important, therefore, that this resource is not damaged by everyday life. People do have aspirations about themselves; they may not express those aspirations in terms of health, but by using other language. These aspirations may be simple ones: of doing a good job at work, having a home in which to bring up their family, to earn sufficient money to have a good and interesting life with sufficient food, warmth and protection. Our aspirations reflect the society in which we live; our needs are those of our society and culture. There needs to be consideration of the environment that people live in, their housing, diet, leisure activities, work. To have people who feel they are healthy in a community must make that community healthy, and give it a strong sense of identity and feeling of being positive and empowered.

The WHO Regional Office for Europe published *Targets for Health for All* (WHO, 1985), arising out of the Alma Ata Conference and Health for All by the Year 2000. The European targets reflect the industrial base of the member countries and focus on three areas: the promotion of lifestyles conducive to health, the reduction of preventable conditions, and the provision of care which is adequate, accessible and acceptable to all.

Defining and measuring health

McDowell and Newell (1987) identify the need for a conceptualisation of terminology in measuring health or its deviations. They argue that any approach to measurement should have as its basis a conceptual framework.

> The conceptual definition of an index relates it to a broader body of theory and shows how the results obtained may be interpreted in the light of that theory. (McDowell and Newell, 1987, p. 23)

The difficulty arises in trying to use the many and various definitions available for use. Hunt *et al.* (1986) identify the three dominant concepts which must be included in studies which address health status, namely health, disease and illness. These writers acknowledge that to decide or describe what health is not is usually greeted with more approval than attempts to describe what health is. They go on to conclude that the presence of health relates to capacities which are social, psychological, physical and functional and in a manner relative to time, place and contemporary technology.

Until approximately the beginning of the nineteenth century, 'health' was seen as soundness of mind, body and spirit (Gott and O'Brien, 1990). The emergence of 'science' brought about a shift towards the delivery of health care based on areas of specialism which are increasingly narrowly defined. There is a need to open wide the debate about health and illness, to listen to what people tell us about their life, their work, their minds and bodies; to use this information in a way that will help them and, it is hoped, enrich their lives, through addressing what they see as their health needs. We need to consider the individual as a whole, and not the parts of a whole. Patrick's story in Box 1.5 illustrates this need.

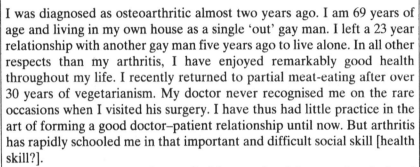

Box 1.5: Patrick

I was diagnosed as osteoarthritic almost two years ago. I am 69 years of age and living in my own house as a single 'out' gay man. I left a 23 year relationship with another gay man five years ago to live alone. In all other respects than my arthritis, I have enjoyed remarkably good health throughout my life. I recently returned to partial meat-eating after over 30 years of vegetarianism. My doctor never recognised me on the rare occasions when I visited his surgery. I have thus had little practice in the art of forming a good doctor–patient relationship until now. But arthritis has rapidly schooled me in that important and difficult social skill [health skill?].

I wake up every morning to find legs and pelvic area that feel and behave as if I've done a week's forced march of fifty miles a day. Joints, muscles and tendons ache, twinge when moved, give way unpredictably, cramp into inflexibility, and reduce you to a doddering stage geriatric. What they don't show you 'on stage' are the grotesque bodily contortions and physical subterfuges needed to continue running your home single-handedly, keep your valued social network operative and maintain yourself financially. Personal hygiene and body care also present problems.

What is even less publicly visible is the psychological culture-shock of rapid disablement – managing pain and the steady depletion of mobility, seeking medical and other help, getting out to the shops, restaurants, cultural events, holidays away, sex, work, money. All these and many other aspects of life suddenly become fraught with new problems. Not just physical problems, but new ways of interpersonal relating and being related to, with attendant psychological demands, worries, hurts and rewards.

Smith (1992) revisits the initial intentions behind the establishment of the NHS. These were:

- to promote the nation's health;
- to ensure the equitable distribution of health care;

- to render the health service accountable to the nation; and
- to invest the activities and development of the NHS with a sense of purpose (Smith, 1992, p. 376).

There is still some way to go in achieving these objectives for health. Smith continues the debate on what is health by identifying the various ways it could be viewed:

- a public resource;
- a commodity for distribution;
- a basic human right.

Smith feels that health is 'contingent on circumstances'; these circumstances could include time, place, events, effects. The definition of health offered by Smith is:

> people are healthy to the extent that they are able to meet their obligations and to enjoy the rewards associated with membership of their community. (Smith, 1992, p. 37).

Smith focuses on the notion of individuality in relationship to health, and feels that strategies developed for health would also need to demonstrate this notion. This is an interesting argument in that his definition of health has elements of collectivism in it. The individual will be able to meet his personal obligations which will maintain the community, allowing for rewards. This seems to suggest a 'systems approach' (Silverman, 1970), the sum of the parts working to achieve the good of the whole. Smith continues this approach by stating that a national strategy for health should be based on a clear national health policy where the importance of health, alongside other important national goals, for example defence, economic growth, education and transport, is clearly identified and stated. This vision needs to be compared to the vision held by people who would be described as reductionist.

Sources of information

The way that we perceive any issue is influenced by the availability of information. This is no different for health. For example, many health statistics do not record ethnicity and this has led to neglect of debate and policy development around the health of people from minority ethnic groups. The main sources used in this book are official statistics, major national surveys, local surveys and personal stories. The purpose of this section is twofold: to give the reader information on the availability and coverage of the sources for follow up in more detail if required; and to review the perspective and assumptions built into the data.

Official statistics

The Decennial Census (OPCS, 1993a). The 1991 Census included a question about ethnicity for the first time (OPCS, 1993b) which has made demographic and health-related analyses possible.

The General Household Survey (GHS) is conducted annually on a large sample of people and covers a wide range of topics including self-assessment of health. Some topics are covered periodically such as chronic illness, alcohol and smoking in the 1992 survey (OPCS, 1992).

The Health Survey for England is carried out annually. Topics covered include: psychosocial wellbeing; general health and use of services and prescribed medicines; physical activity, eating habits and obesity; smoking and alcohol consumption.

Major national surveys

The Health and Lifestyle Survey (Cox *et al.*, 1993) was conducted in 1984/85 with 9,003 respondents who were followed up seven years later and a total of 5,532 of the original sample were resurveyed. It is one of the very few longitudinal health surveys carried out in Britain. Topics covered include: physical health; psychological health; lifestyle; social factors. There have been two major reviews of health using secondary data which provide very useful sources: 'The health of adult Britain' (ONS, 1997) and 'The health of our children' (ONS, 1995).

Health service reports

The annual report of the Chief Medical Officer, 'On the state of the public health', provides a useful review of the year and usually includes a chapter on a special topic. It was the 1992 report which had the chapter 'Health of men' which provided an important official boost to the subject (DOH, 1992).

The annual reports of Directors of Public Health of district health authorities provide useful overviews of health in their district (see, for example, Birmingham Health Authority, 1995). For the last few years these reports have been closely patterned on the key areas and targets of the Health of the Nation strategy. Unfortunately the reports of the Regional Directors of Public Health (see, for example, NHSE-WM, 1994) have been discontinued when regional health authorities were abolished and replaced by regional offices of the NHS Executive.

Personal stories

Official statistics and reports provide information about aggregates of the population, usually at a particular point in time. We also need to hear the direct experience of boys and men in order to understand how their masculinities develop over time, and how they experience the dynamic interaction in their lives of a multitude of factors and influences which cannot be captured in cross-sectional surveys. Since the late 1970s there has been a considerable output of personal stories by women but much less by men. In this book we have drawn on this limited literature where available; we see that a major requirement for progress of men's health is to develop a much wider selection of personal stories which will express something of the diversity of men's lives.

Health policy

Public health and health at work

The history of occupational disease and ill health was documented by Ramazzini in 1713 (English translation, 1964) and later by Thackrah (1832), and still this history does not seem to have an effect on policy developers' perception of the need for health care in the workplace. This is further removed from the provision of health care nationally by the definite policy decision to distance health care at work from health care generally (Townsend and Davidson, 1982). Occupational health is not seen as part of the public health. In 1985 the Secretary of State for Health established a committee of enquiry into the 'future development of public health function' with the following terms of reference:

> To consider the future development of the public health function, including the control of communicable diseases and the speciality of community medicine, following the introduction of general management into the Hospital and Community Health Services, and recognising a continued need for improvements in effectiveness and efficiency: and to make recommendations as soon as possible, and no later than December 1986. (DOH, 1988, p. 26)

The committee membership included a wide range of people concerned with the health of the public. This committee defined public health as:

> The art and science of preventing disease, prolonging life and promoting health through the organised efforts of society. (DOH, 1988, p. 26)

This review was the first comprehensive review of the public health since the Royal Sanitary Commission of 1871. This was an ideal opportunity to review the health of the public in its widest sense. The opportunity was not taken up. The recommendations centred on the activities within the National Health Service; reminding health authorities of their responsibilities for health, that public health doctors should be part of the decision-making machinery of the authority (general management), that an annual report should be produced on the state of the health of the district, and that a central unit be set up at the Department of Health to monitor the health of the population from a national perspective.

This was a lost opportunity to produce a more integrated approach to promoting health. Health at work will be a main focus in Chapter 5. This serious omission has to some extent been rectified by the government publication *Our Healthier Nation* (DOH, 1998a). This document put the workplace as a key target area for health interventions together with schools and communities.

Outline

We have set out the rationale for the book in this chapter. Figure 1.1 shows how the chapters develop our ideas through the book leading to the summary and recommendations in Chapter 9.

Chapters 2, 3 and 4 describe what we know and what we don't know about men's health. Chapter 2 uses qualitative and quantitative information to provide an overview of what is known about demography, mortality and morbidity. There are comparisons by class and ethnicity and some international comparisons. Chapter 3 reviews the socialisation of males from infancy to manhood and how the different aspects of masculinity develop. This forms the basis for Chapter 4 where we describe and attempt to understand health and illness behaviour.

Chapters 5 and 6 focus on men's health in the workplace. The subjective importance of work to men's identity and the objective influences of the work environment on health are the subject of Chapter 5 which concentrates on men in the age range 16–59 years. The workplace also offers an important opportunity for getting health messages and health services to men. Unemployment and non-work are also considered in this chapter. Chapter 6 is based on original research carried out in a number of workplaces in the West Midlands to find out what men and women thought about their health. It shows, therefore, the diversity of men's and women's experiences and attitudes.

Chapters 7 and 8 examine national and local policy initiatives and debate how these might be taken forward. Chapter 7 describes a number of strategic case studies from European countries and Australia, and discusses how to take policy forward and whether there should be an explicit national policy for men's health. Chapter 8 looks below the national level, mainly in Britain but with some examples from other countries, at how initiatives for men's health have developed both within the health service and independently.

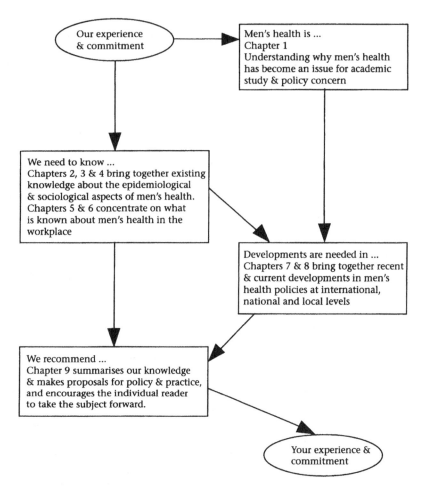

Figure 1.1   How the themes are developed in the chapters.

Finally, Chapter 9 presents a mapping of how the ideas through the book are related including what we do and what we don't know, and summarises the arguments for developing men's health. It concludes by explaining what the authors intend to do in the future.

Summary

In this chapter we have described why men's health has emerged as a public issue in the last decade, partly due to recognition that men's health has been neglected compared with the increasing attention to other stratification since the Health of the Nation strategy was published (DOH, 1992), and partly due to the unprecedented rise in young male suicides and mortality from HIV/AIDS. We have compared the development of interest in men's health with that in women's health which arose earlier and largely due to social change and political pressures from outside the health service. We recommend that the reader reflects on his or her personal experiences of men's health, as the authors have done, in order to maintain a fruitful balance between the concrete and abstract. Finally, we have provided an outline of subjects of the chapters and how they are related in an overall structure.

Further reading

Bruckenwell, P., Jackson, D., Luck, M., Wallace, J. and Watts, J. (1995) *The Crisis in Men's Health*. Community Health UK, Bath.

This book contains a selection of accounts by five men of health related experiences in their lives. In most cases there is a connection to socialisation in childhood.

Doyal, L. (1995) *What Makes Women Sick. Gender and the Political Economy of Health*. Macmillan, Basingstoke.

This book is valuable because it establishes the links between women's health and the political economy and puts this analysis into an international context. Much work is needed before it will be possible to write such a book about men's health.

Phillips, A. and Rakusen, J. (1996, revised edition) *The New Our Bodies Ourselves*. Penguin, Harmondsworth.

This book is a classic which sets an enviable standard for providing a mass of information in an accessible form, and it is inspiring because it shows how a large scale collaborative effort can be effective.

Chapter 2
Overview of Male Health

In this chapter we:

- show that male birth rates have been consistently higher than female and, consequently, males outnumber females in the population up to the age of 50;
- show that life expectancy has increased dramatically in the last 150 years but the gap in life expectancy between females and males has increased;
- show that the life expectancy of the civilian population increased more rapidly in the two decades which included the First and Second World Wars;
- show that as a result of differential patterns of migration, minority ethnic groups have age and sex distributions that differ considerably from the white population;
- argue that the increase in male mortality rates in Eastern Europe cannot be explained by lifestyle or environmental pollution and is most likely due to a crisis in masculinity.

Introduction

In this chapter our aim is to provide a statistical profile of the male population and of male mortality and morbidity. We shall compare this, where appropriate, with female mortality and morbidity. We shall then try to explain these data in Chapters 4, 5 and 6 using the social perspectives on masculinities to be developed in Chapter 3.

The age–sex distribution of the population is determined by birth rates and death rates, but it is also important to analyse this by ethnicity because the migration patterns of the minority ethnic groups are diverse. We would expect that ethnic disadvantage will affect health.

The profiles of mortality and life expectancy since the mid nineteenth century and the trends therein throw light on sex differences and the impact of social change including the two World Wars.

We undertake international comparisons of some of these indicators.

This will show how Britain's place has changed in international 'league tables'. Further clues about the effect of social factors on health come from a comparison of data from Western and Eastern European countries in the period when the Iron Curtain came down.

Demography

Age–sex profile

The numbers of males and females in 10-year age groups are shown in Table 2.1. There are more males than females in the younger age groups. Forecasts of the numbers of men in the 20–29 and 30–39 age groups based on the numbers of births and deaths for these cohorts suggest under-enumeration in the 1991 Census. It is thought that there were more men than women in these age groups who did not respond because they wished to avoid the 'poll tax', now replaced by the council tax. This 'under coverage' was estimated to be 'around 9% for men in their twenties' (OPCS, 1994, p. 5).

Table 2.1   Population of Great Britain by age and sex.

age	males	females	ratio m:f
0–9	3,295,679	3,143,172	1.05
10–19	3,168,143	3,024,857	1.05
20–29	3,802,340	3,899,944	0.97
30–39	3,446,271	3,484,619	0.99
40–49	3,361,529	3,374,209	1.00
50–59	2,635,823	2,650,903	0.99
60–69	2,388,626	2,660,595	0.90
70–79	1,521,409	2,156,325	0.71
80+	563,173	1,312,660	0.43
Total	24,182,993	25,707,284	0.94

Source: OPCS (1993a) Table 2, p. 64

Birth rates

Table 2.2 shows the number of live births at 10 year intervals since 1950. During the whole period there are between 5% and 6% more boys born than girls. This difference is consistent across industrialised countries. The higher conception rate for boys would appear to be a device of nature to compensate for the fact boys are more vulnerable than girls in the womb and have a higher infant mortality rate (Barker, 1994).

Table 2.2 Live births since 1950 by sex, England and Wales.

Year	Males	Females	Ratio M-F
1950	358,715	338,312	1.06
1960	404,150	380,855	1.06
1970	403,371	381,115	1.06
1980	335,954	320,280	1.05
1990	361,412	344,728	1.05

Source: ONS (1995) Tables 1.4 and 1.5, pp. 6, 7.

Ethnicity

The age distributions of the male population by ethnicity, grouped as white, black and Asian, show considerable differences; as in Figure 2.1. The main difference is that there are proportionately more men in the 'working age group' (16–59) and fewer men in the older age group (60+) in both the black and Asian populations compared with the white population due to the patterns of migration.

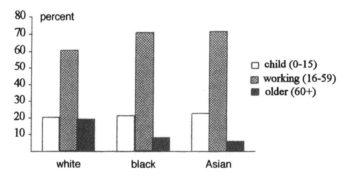

Figure 2.1 Proportions of males in ethnic groups by age. *Source: OPCS (1993b) Table 6, pp. 496, 498.*

Migration is an important and dynamic factor in the make-up of the minority ethnic groups. In the working age group, 16–59, the proportion who were born in Britain varies from 53% for Caribbeans to 13% for Bangladeshis; whereas for children, 0–15, the proportions are 96% for Caribbeans and 78% for Bangladeshis (Modood *et al.*, 1997, Table 2.2, p. 21).

Marital status

The marital status among whites and the minority ethnic groups except for Caribbeans is roughly similar. For whites and Asian groups the proportions of adults under 60 who are single varies between 23% and 29%, and the proportions who are married or living as married varies from 69% to 75%. However, for Caribbeans the proportion who are single is 41% and the proportion who are married or living as married is 49% (see Modood *et al.*, 1997, Table 2.4, p. 24).

In the 1991 Census the proportion of mixed-ethnicity partnerships was only 1% of the population as a whole, showing that very few white people have a partner from a minority ethnic group. The PSI survey in 1994 showed that about 20% of Caribbean adults were married or living as married to a white partner, 17% of Chinese, 4% of Indians and African Asians, and only 1% of Pakistanis and Bangladeshis (Modood *et al.*, 1997, p. 30). Attitudes towards mixed-ethnicity partnerships will be discussed in Chapter 3.

Life expectancy and mortality

Historical profile

Life expectancy has increased dramatically since the middle of the nine-teenth century, by 32 years for males from 41 to 73, and by 36 years for females from 43 to 79, as shown in Figure 2.2. The difference in life expectancy between males and females has thus increased from two to six years over this period. This has, of course, huge implications for health and social services with the need to shift emphasis to quality of life and main-taining independence during the later years in contrast to saving and

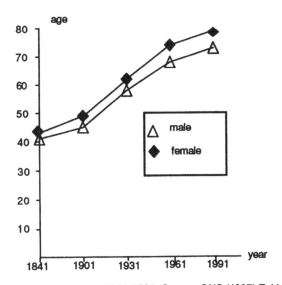

Figure 2.2 Life expectancy by sex 1841–1991. *Source: ONS (1997) Table 3.3, p. 20.*

extending life which has been the emphasis for most of the twentieth century.

Mortality by age

The decrease in mortality during the 150 year period under examination has taken place mainly in the younger age groups; for those who had survived to 55 there was little reduction until the 1920s; and for those who survived until 75 the reduction in mortality has been even more recent, as shown in Figure 2.3.

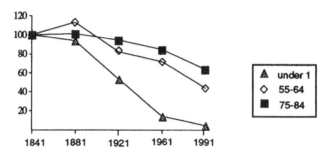

Figure 2.3   Trends in mortality in three age groups. *Source: ONS (1997) Table 3.4, p. 23.*

Male and female death rates by age

Although the absolute death rates have declined for both sexes and all age groups as shown above, the ratio of male to female death rates varies greatly over this period by age. Figure 2.4 shows this ratio for three age groups. For deaths under one year old there has been little change in the ratio during the whole of this period. For young adults, however, there has been a large increase in the ratio of male to female deaths: with the ratio for the age group 20–24 years old increasing from 105 in 1841 to more than double, 261, in 1991. For the older age groups the ratio has increased over the period, but not to the same extent.

Life expectancy and inequalities

Wilkinson (1996) has shown that the life expectancy for males and females in England and Wales has increased in every decade in the twentieth century, see Figure 2.5. But by far the greatest increases in life expectancy (excluding military deaths) came in the two decades which included World Wars I and II and which saw a return to full employment and a dramatic

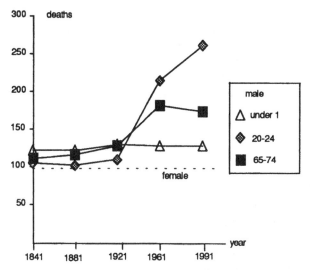

Figure 2.4 Ratio of male to female death rates, 1841–1991. *Source: ONS (1997) Table 3.4, p. 23.*

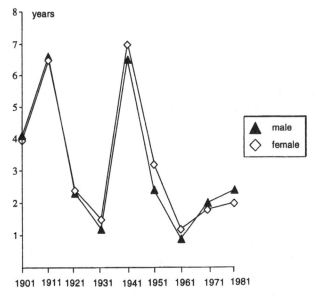

Figure 2.5 Increases in male and female life expectancy, 1901–1990. *Source: Wilkinson (1996) Table 6.2, p. 114.*

narrowing of income differentials. This suggests that in developed countries further increases in life expectancy are not dependent on increases in national wealth, as measured by GDP, but are dependent upon increases in 'social capital', whether people feel positive about their relative position and value in society. Income inequality is one measure of social capital.

There is further discussion of the hypothesis of the relationship between health and social capital in Chapter 4.

Class

The Black report

There is a long tradition of analysis of mortality data by social class which has been carried out since the nineteenth century, but the heightening of debate from the point of view of policy and research occurred with the publication of the Black report by the Research Working Group on Inequalities in Health which was appointed in 1977 by David Ennals, then Secretary of State for Health in the Labour government (Townsend and Davidson, 1982). The report was published in August 1980 by which time Patrick Jenkin was Secretary of State in a Conservative government.

In January 1986 Dr David Player, Director of the Health Education Council, appointed Margaret Whitehead to assess the progress on the 37 recommendations in the Black report. This report was published on 24 March 1987 (Whitehead, 1988) and the government decided to abolish the HEC on 31 March 1987. According to some MPs the HEC was abolished because it campaigned too vigorously against the tobacco, alcohol and sugar industries which contributed large amounts of money to Conservative Party funds.

The Black report demonstrated in some detail based on the available data at that time that there are considerable inequalities in health by social class, gender, region, and ethnicity; that there were inequalities in the availability and use of services; and that there were considerable international differences and longitudinal trends, especially infant mortality.

The Research Working Group on Inequalities in Health examined various possible explanations and concluded that while cultural and genetic explanations have some relevance the major factor is likely to be 'materialist':

> the more diffuse consequences of the class structure: poverty, work conditions ... and deprivation in its various forms in the home and immediate environment, at work, in education and the upbringing of children and more generally in family and social life. (Townsend and Davidson, 1982, p. 126)

The recommendations concentrated on three main areas:

- children should have a better start in life;
- helping disabled people, including the elderly, to reduce their need for institutional care;
- encouraging good health through preventive and educational action.

The principal aim of the Health Divide report (Whitehead, 1988) was to examine how far the recommendations of the Black report had been implemented. The report concluded that:

> The response to the recommendations has been characterised by a lack of action, particularly at national and central level. No unifying lead has been taken to guide and motivate a response which would have translated recommendations into action. (Townsend and Davidson, 1982, p. 355)

A paper by Davey Smith *et al.* (1990) provided a summary of research on inequalities at that time. In terms of international comparisons there had been: 'Widening of inequalities over this period [1970s] [which] was noticeable only for England and Wales.' They also criticised the emphasis of research in the previous decade:

> the neglect of the area that the Black report described as materialist should not continue . . . studies . . . seem to be focused on the much investigated topics of lifestyles and selection.

Three of the themes from the Black report and *The Health Divide* are still relevant for this book:

- analysis of mortality between social classes, over time and international comparisons;
- the debate about explanations for inequalities;
- whether national policy should be and can be effective.

The two additional themes which we develop in this book are:

- describing sex differences in health, morbidity and mortality; and
- explaining the differences in terms of gender socialisation.

Defining class

The long experience of defining social class by occupation, the Registrar General classification, has been used in every decennial census and in birth and death registration. There has, however, been increasing criticism that the classification is based on the assumption that the head of household is male and has a stable full-time job for life. None of these assumptions remains true: there are many households with a single female head; unemployment is widespread, part-time work is increasing, and there is the shift from industrial manual work to technical and service occupations.

These difficulties have been more significant for women and for young people.

The recent authoritative review of health inequalities (Drever and Whitehead, 1997) provides an excellent survey of data about inequalities in mortality by social class and a more limited survey of inequalities in morbidity. It also examines the sensitivity of the conclusions about inequalities to the revisions in classification of occupations, and explores the use of an alternative social classification based on housing tenure and access to a car. These methodological issues are important in order that conclusions are agreed to be sufficiently robust to feed into policy making.

Inequalities and class

In the previous sections in this chapter we have examined trends in national mortality and life expectancy over long periods of time. However, the various authors in Drever and Whitehead (1997) show that trends can be detected over much shorter periods. For example, Hattersley (1997) shows that male life expectancy at birth over the 20-year period 1972–91 increased for all social classes, but the gap between the life expectancy of classes I and II combined and classes IV and V combined increased during this period. In fact life expectancy for class IV/V increased during the first half of the decade but then stayed stationary for the second half of the decade. One of the conclusions from this analysis – that changes in male life expectancy by social class can be detected in such a short period – is unexpected and is an important contribution to the emerging understanding of the relationship between mortality and social capital for each sex. This is discussed further in Chapter 4.

Smith and Harding (1997) examine the effect of using an alternative social classification based on housing tenure and access to cars. The is particularly relevant for women and older people who cannot always be classified by occupation. Thus of the 1971 Longitudinal Study (LS) cohort of women aged over 65 years, 53% could be classified by occupational class but 95% by tenure and car access, whereas the proportions were 85% and 96% respectively for men.

For men in the 1971 LS the mortality gap between those who were more or less advantaged by housing tenure or access to a car narrowed in the age range 35–44 and widened in the age range 45–64.

Ethnicity

The health of people from minority ethnic groups has tended to be seen from two perspectives: (a) presenting unusual diseases which are the subject for biomedical research; (b) the difficulties of black and Asian people adjusting to the prevailing white norms (Ahmad, 1993). In order to move beyond these perspectives which see minority ethnic groups as passive and problematic, it is necessary to understand something about definitions of ethnicity, demography and ethnic disadvantage. Fortunately, the results of the recent Fourth National Survey of Ethnic Minorities are now available. This survey was undertaken in 1994 by the Policy Studies Institute (PSI) and Social and Community Planning Research (SPCR) (Modood *et al.*, 1997). A nationally representative sample of 5196 people of Caribbean and Asian origin were interviewed in detail, together with a comparison sample of 2867 white people. The survey covered education, employment, housing, health, racial harassment and ethnic identity.

Defining ethnicity

Defining ethnicity has always been problematic: proponents have argued for skin colour (relevant particularly for racial harassment), religion (but people may change or leave a religion), cultural and community links (but these can be difficult to define and fuzzy and change over time), and place of birth (only relevant for older people who migrated here, increasingly younger people tend to have been born in Britain). In the 1991 Census it was decided that people should make their own decision, see Figure 2.6.

Please tick the appropriate box

white ☐
black-Caribbean ☐
black-African ☐
black-other ☐
please describe

If you are descended from more than one ethnic or racial group, please tick the group to which you consider you belong, or tick the 'Any other ethnic group' box and describe your ancestry in the space provided

Indian ☐
Pakistani ☐
Bangladeshi ☐
Chinese ☐
any other ethnic group ☐
please describe

Figure 2.6 Self-definition of ethnic group in 1991 Census. *Source: OPCS (1993b) Question 11.*

This includes both skin colour 'white' and 'black' and country of origin, 'Indian', 'Pakistani', 'Bangladeshi', and 'Chinese'. The Fourth National Survey used both the census self-definition together with a question about 'family origins'. The two definitions were largely equivalent. We will, therefore, rely on the 1991 Census definition in this book to classify populations.

It is important for health workers to understand in more depth about culture and identity as this will affect how masculinities develop for men and how they respond to health and illness. For the South Asians, Modood *et al.* (1997) suggest seven indicators of identity: three behavioural, clothes, religion and language; and four attitudinal, about marriage, description, self-identity and school. There are considerable differences by subgroup, by gender and by age, see Table 2.3. For all four subgroups men wear Asian clothes less than women, with African Asian men having the lowest proportion. Younger men, 16–34, wear Asian clothes less than older men.

Table 2.3 The wearing of Asian clothes by men.

| | *percentages* | | | |
	Indian	African Asian	Pakistani	Bangladeshi
Always	6	1	7	7
Sometimes	51	41	77	69
Never	43	58	16	24
16–34 year-olds				
Always	2	1	1	4
Sometimes	47	37	79	61
Never	52	62	20	34

Source: Modood et al. (1997) Table 9.31, p. 327.

The involvement of parents in choice of marriage partner has decreased. When analysed by religion there has been the generation decrease, see Table 2.4, and for all ages and for Hindus and Muslims the parental involvement is higher for women than men. The only exception is for Sikh

Table 2.4 Parental involvement in choice of marriage partner by sex, religion and age.

| | *Hindu* | | *Sikh* | | *Muslim* | |
	Men	Women	Men	Women	Men	Women
50+ years old	50	74	72	86	62	87
35–49 years old	21	51	49	77	59	78
16–34 years old	18	20	41	27	49	67

Source: Modood et al. (1997) Table 9.23, p. 318.

men where the influence of parents has decreased for women from 77%, for 35–49 years, to 27%, for 16–34 years, whereas for men there has been a much slower decrease from 49%, for 35–49 years, to 41%, for 16–34 years.

Ethnic disadvantage

The advantage of having the three previous comparable national surveys, carried out in 1966 (Daniel, 1968), 1974 (Smith, 1977) and 1982 (Brown, 1984) is that comparisons can be made and assessments of progress or regression in socio-economic conditions. Health was only introduced in the fourth 1994 survey (Modood *et al.*, 1997), but as we have already commented socio-economic conditions have a major, perhaps primary, influence on health.

The first survey in 1966 (Daniel, 1968) showed that for West Indians migration was almost complete and there were approximately the same numbers of men and women. However, for Asians only about a third of migration had been completed from India and Pakistan; very few African Asians or Bangladeshis (from East Pakistan at the time) had come; and there were far more men than women. Employment was almost entirely in manual labour. Housing was mainly in poor quality private rented accommodation in inner cities areas that whites were vacating.

By the time of the second survey in 1974 (Smith, 1977), migration of the Asians had continued with more emphasis on women and children, but men still outnumbered women. There had been some movement into skilled manual employment, but very few had been able to enter white-collar jobs, despite suitable education and qualifications. There were significant changes in housing: for Caribbeans, half were owner-occupiers, a quarter council house tenants, and a quarter in private rented accommodation; three-quarters of Asians were owner-occupiers. When asked if they thought that life had improved for their ethnic groups in the preceding five years, there were more Asians and Caribbeans who agreed than disagreed.

The third survey in 1982 (Brown, 1984), took place during a major recession and reduction in jobs in labour-intensive manufacturing. Unemployment was higher than among the white population for all ethnic minority groups except Indian and African Asian men. Self-employment had increased significantly among Asians. When the same question was asked about whether life had improved for their ethnic group in the preceding five years, the responses were much more pessimistic than in 1974.

The most recent fourth survey in 1994 widened the topics covered. A major finding was that the differences between the minority ethnic groups had increased: Pakistanis and Bangladeshis were in serious poverty, with expected impacts on their health (see Chapter 4); unemployment for men and women was very high, and those who were employed were in the lowest income jobs; Caribbeans and Indians were less disadvantaged than the Pakistanis and Bangladeshis; Chinese and African Asians were on a similar level to whites – on some indicators they were ahead.

Racial harassment

Overall 13% of people from minority ethnic groups reported that they had been subjected to some form of racial harassment in the previous twelve months. More males (15%) than females (11%) reported harassment. Harassment was highest for Chinese (16%) and lowest for Bangladeshis (9%). Younger people in the age range 16–44 reported more harassment (15%) than people aged 45+ (9%). The extent to which racial harassment affects health will be discussed in Chapter 4.

The Irish in Britain

The Irish form the largest minority ethnic group in Britain and experience inequality and discrimination. Nevertheless, there has been little discussion about their needs in the race relations debates nor action to redress these problems. A survey commissioned by the Commission For Racial Equality (CRE) has found:

> The Irish are excluded from consideration in these [race relations] terms because they are white and the dominant paradigm for understanding racism in Britain today is constructed on the basis of a black-white dichotomy. (Hickman and Walter, 1997, 7)

Resulting from the report, the CRE has recommended that the next national census in 2001 should include an Irish category in the ethnic origin question, and that all ethnic monitoring systems, which would include NHS ethnic monitoring, should include an Irish category (CRE, 1997).

The health of Irish-born men is a matter of concern. They form the only migrant group whose mortality is higher in Britain than in their country of origin. This disadvantage appears to be continuing into the second generation born in Britain who have higher mortality from all cancers for men in the age range 15–64, and the higher rates cannot be explained by social class differences.

Poverty, mortality and hospital admissions

An extensive analysis of the relationship between poverty, sex and mortality and hospital admissions is provided in the 1994 Report of the Regional Director of Public Health (NHSE-WM, 1994).

Mortality

Figure 2.7 shows that mortality increases with poverty, represented by the Townsend level, for all age groups except 15–24.

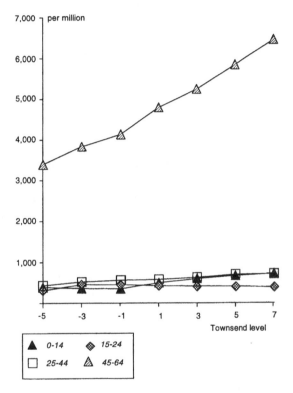

Figure 2.7 Mortality and poverty by age. *Source: West Midlands Cancer Intelligence Unit adapted from NHSE-WM (1994).*

In the West Midlands, generally speaking the poorer the area that someone lives in the more likely they are to die as a child. The death rates in the poorest areas are almost twice those in the most affluent areas. But one of the main causes of death in childhood, cancer, is more common among children from higher social class families.

The death rate for males, 15–24 years, is more than twice that for females in this age group. There is no clear trend for deaths related to poverty in this age group, unlike the younger and older age groups.

The death rates for males are considerably higher than for females in the 25–44 age group. The slope of the male line with poverty is steeper than the female line. Whatever it is that leads to higher death rates in men is less prevalent in the richer areas. If the higher death rate is associated with more risk taking behaviour then it seems that richer men are more careful.

Death rates for men 45–64 are higher than for women, and the slope of the relationship with the Townsend score is much steeper for men than women. Death rates for men in the most deprived areas are much higher than in the better off areas.

The relationship of death rates with poverty in the 65+ age group is much less clear than for the younger age groups. For men there is a very slight increase but not for women.

Hospital admissions

Poverty is also associated with an increasing risk of hospital admission. Even though children from the poorer areas are more likely to be admitted to hospital, it still does not prevent them from dying.

For adolescents, 10–19 years, even when admissions related to childbirth are removed, females have a slightly higher hospital admission rate than males. There is only a slight increase with poverty for men in this age group.

In the middle years, 45–64 years, female admission rates are higher than the male rates, but the lines have similar slopes. This suggests that the relationship between poverty and hospital admission may be similar for men and women. This is not the case for the relationship between death and poverty in this age group.

In the retirement age, 65+ years, admission rates for men are slightly lower than for women, but there is a clear increase in admissions with poverty. This may be because there are more women in the very elderly age groups, 75+ years, who live alone and are more likely to be admitted to hospital.

International comparisons

There is considerable value in making comparisons with other countries, particularly other European countries with similar levels of socio-economic development. Comparison of demographic and health statistics can lead to pressure on politicians and senior health service officials of the 'we ought to do better' variety, which is one way of attacking complacency of the 'we have the best health service in the world' variety. But, more importantly, it may help us to look behind the statistics for causal relations between the social and economic factors which we cover in the next chapter.

Infant mortality in Europe

Comparison of infant mortality rates (IMR) between countries of the European Union over the 20-year period of 1971 to 1991 shows that all the countries have made considerable reductions in IMR and that the range has narrowed. In 1971 the highest male IMR was Portugal (55.0 deaths per 1000 live births) and the lowest was the Netherlands (14.0); by 1991 the highest IMR was Portugal (12.2) and the lowest were the Netherlands and West Germany (both 7.7), as shown in Figure 2.8.

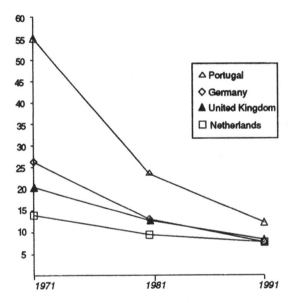

Figure 2.8   Male infant mortality in selected European countries, 1971–1991. *Source: ONS (1995) Table 6.14, pp. 79–80.*

The ratio of male to female deaths remained remarkably stable at 1.3 for all countries over this 20-year period despite the considerable reductions in both female and male IMR.

Western and eastern Europe compared

Watson (1995) has compared mortality by gender in western and eastern European countries between 1970 and 1990. In 1970 male mortality rates (MMR) were lower in a number of eastern European countries than some western European countries; for example the MMR for East Germany was lower than for West Germany. Between 1970 and 1990 MMR reduced for all western European countries and increased for all eastern European countries as shown in Figure 2.9. Further, the MMR for former Yugoslavia, which could be considered to be politically and geographically on the boundary between western and eastern Europe, stayed the same.

In particular, for men who were not married, divorced or separated, death rates increased rapidly. In Poland death rates by age for married men changed little between 1970 and 1988 whereas the death rates for divorced men increased greatly, see Figure 2.10.

Between 1970 and 1990 female mortality rates (FMR) improved in all western and eastern European countries except Hungary. In 1990 the FMR for some eastern European countries was better than some western European countries, Scotland having one of the highest FMRs.

In contrast to these statistics for adult men and women (aged 25–64), death rates for males and females aged 1–24 continued to fall in eastern Europe; in some countries, Czechoslovakia, for example, this was as rapid as for western European countries.

The increase in MMR for adult males in eastern Europe, in contrast to adult females and young males and young females, cannot be explained by changes in behavioural risk factors such as smoking, diet and alcohol. Nor can the increases be explained by environmental factors such as pollution. The argument that these differences can be explained in terms of the relationship between health and social capital is taken up in Chapter 4, Health Inequalities and Social Capital.

Summary

Statistics of mortality and life expectancy have mainly shown consistent long-term trends in reduction (mortality) and increase (life expectancy). The relative advantage of females over males has shown remarkable consistency over the past 150 years. The main recent deviation has been for young men, where the disadvantage compared with young women has worsened significantly in the past 30 years. Comparisons with other European countries show similar trends, except that eastern European indicators have worsened, especially for men.

The evidence is strong that health is strongly linked to social capital measured by income inequalities. Men are less able to utilise family and social networks and are more affected by social deprivation and unemployment. This offers a likely explanation as to why it is the deaths of young men in the western European countries and single men in the eastern European countries which run counter to the long-term trends in reduction in mortality.

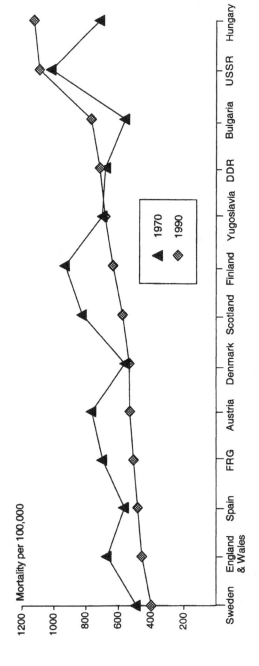

Figure 2.9 Male mortality in Europe, selected countries 1970 and 1990. *Source: Watson (1995) Figure 1, p. 925.*

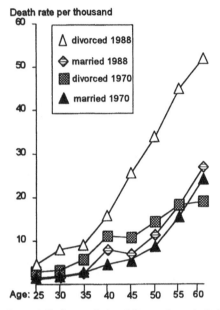

Figure 2.10 Changes in mortality for married and divorced men in Poland between 1970 and 1988. *Source: Watson (1995) Figure 7, p. 931.*

Further reading

Modood *et al.* (1997) *Ethnic Minorities in Britain*. Policy Studies Institute, London. This survey provides an essential source of information about ethnic minorities, including demography, employment and health. It provides résumés and comparisons with the preceding three national surveys which were carried out at approximately ten-year intervals.

ONS (1997) *The Health of Adult Britain 1841–1994*. The Stationery Office, London. This book provides a mine of information about demography, mortality and morbidity over the 150-year period covered. It provides a high standard of presentation and explanation.

Watson, P. (1995) Explaining rising mortality among men in EEastern Europe, *Social Science Med.*, **41**, 7, 923–34. This journal article shows how female and male mortality in eastern European countries compares with western European countries, and explains the increasing mortality of men in eastern Europe in terms of their lack of social capital.

Wilkinson, R. (1996) *Unhealthy Societies*. Routledge, London. Wilkinson provides the first major progress of the debate about health inequalities. The emphasis on the relationship of health to social capital is important, although he does not take account of gender differences in building and using social capital.

Chapter 3

Gender and Masculinities

In this chapter we:

- clarify the differences between 'sex' and 'gender';
- review childhood influences on boys and how they are socialised to become men, including what is known about the influence of present and absent fathers;
- argue that masculinity is not unchanging nor is it an internally consistent set of relationships and practices, therefore it is more fruitful to discuss 'masculinities';
- show that masculinities are strongly reinforced by state violence, domestic violence and sport;
- explore how the perspectives of ethnicity and racism, ability and 'disabilism', and class intersect with masculinities;
- debate the question 'Can men change?'.

Introduction

> **Real Men (Part 1)**
>
> Real men keep fit
> Real men don't give a shit
>
> Real men beat the wife
> Real men get life
>
> Real men don't bathe
> Real men own a lathe
>
> Real men speak plain
> Real men like John Wayne
>
> Real men don't hurt
> Real men like a bit of skirt
>
> Real men work the rigs
> Real men live in digs
>
> Dick Leith, 1998

In this chapter our aim is to develop an analysis of gender with particular reference to the way in which boys and men are socialised. Our understanding of 'masculinities' in this chapter is intended to form a platform for the analysis which follows in Chapters 4, 5 and 6 of the patterns of mortality and morbidity which have been described in Chapter 2.

Since the second wave of feminism in the USA and Britain in the 1970s there has been extensive analysis of gender and the socialisation of women and much descriptive writing of girls' and women's experiences, but far less about boys and men. We try to make clear where there is an absence of reliable data and we have to rely on speculation or hearsay evidence.

A considerable part of this chapter is taken up with issues of definition of terms including 'sex' and 'gender', and 'masculinity' and 'masculinities'. Clear definitions are needed to avoid later confusion when interpreting empirical information on behaviour and attitudes, and the links to health and ill health.

We try to maintain a balance and draw links between an understanding of the diversity of men, avoiding the trap of assuming an essentialist homogenous nature for men, and the social perspectives of class, ethnicity and ability. This has to be a preliminary attempt because of the paucity of empirical data and analyses. Nevertheless we believe that this does advance our understanding and can lead to some practical policies and programs which are considered in Chapters 7 and 8.

Finally, we try to answer the question 'Can men change?'.

Why does gender matter?

In his Annual Report for 1992, the Chief Medical Officer devoted a chapter to the 'Health of Men'. After an extensive review of data on mortality and morbidity, there is a final short section 'Improving the health of men' in which it is acknowledged that:

> Gender differences in mortality and morbidity undoubtedly exist: but what are they caused by and what can be done about them? There is increasing evidence that many of the patterns observed stem from differences in health-related behaviour, which may be influenced by the knowledge, attitudes and beliefs of men. (DOH, 1993, p.105)

We need to understand more clearly how men develop this knowledge and these attitudes and beliefs. It seems likely that they are developed very early in the upbringing of babies, and boys (and girls). So we need to look at the formation of gender and masculinity (and femininity). From the point of view of our knowledge of health and masculinity, there are large gaps:

> '... until recently researchers tended to equate the study of gender and health to studies of women's health and illness...' (Sabo and Gordon, 1995, p. 4).

Source materials on men's health and gender in terms of analyses and debate, surveys and personal stories are not abundant.

We need to understand more clearly how power and resources, which include health, are controlled and distributed in society. In their influential book, *The Policy Process in the Modern Capitalist State*, Ham and Hill (1993) acknowledge that most of the analysis has been in terms of class.

> ... other forms of stratification, particularly stratification in terms of gender and ethnicity, may be significant for the distribution of power ... we have chosen to focus upon the class analysis associated with Marxism, in the absence of a literature which relates these other forms of stratification to the policy process in general. (Ham and Hill 1993, p.34)

Feminist analysis has begun to consider capitalism and social policy in terms of gender with the emphasis on different forms of femininity but a single homogeneous form of masculinity. Williams (1989) reviews the different feminist critiques: libertarian, liberal, welfare, radical, socialist and black. These can be interpreted as representing the interests of different groups of women. For men, there has been little analysis of the experience and interests of different groups, especially those 'subordinated' or 'marginalised' such as homeless, mentally ill, and disabled men.

Sex and gender

Definitions

The difference between 'sex' and 'gender' has been made clear by Ann Oakley:

> 'Sex' is a biological term: 'gender' a psychological and cultural one. Common sense suggests that they are merely two ways of looking at the same division and that someone who belongs to, say, the female sex will automatically belong to the corresponding (feminine) gender. In reality this is not so. To be a man or woman, a boy or girl, is as much a function of dress, gesture, occupation, social network and personality, as it is of possessing a particular set of genitals. (Oakley, 1972, p.158)

How the genders develop

It seems that these patterns which are summarised under the two genders of masculine and feminine begin to be developed and inculcated into males and females at very early ages.

> By age 3, children of both sexes have developed their core gender identities
> as well as their understanding that gender is constant and they can compe-
> tently classify gender-related characteristics. (Stillion, 1995, p. 57)

Cuddling, tone of voice, colour of clothes, choice of toys are all influenced
by the sex of the baby and thus serve to define and reinforce the gendered
patterns of behaviour.

Recently *The Hite Report On the Family* (Hite, 1994) shows how these
patterns are developed in families. Strong as the prevailing patterns are, we
should be aware that the patterns do vary, so we should not become
entrenched in an essentialist view that this is inevitable. Although the
evidence from the *Hite Report* is illuminating we should bear in mind also
that the sample of respondents was approximately 50% from the United
States, 35% from the UK and Europe, and the remaining 15% from many
other countries. We should use the evidence with care, and before reaching
conclusions should try to check it out with local studies.

The concept of 'the family' is one that needs careful elucidation. The
norm of the family as a married couple with children carries political weight
and has been used by both politicians and the press to criticise parents and
children who do not live in this conventional unit and to blame them for
delinquency and other social problems. This is despite the fact that the
evidence shows that few adults or children do live in the conventional
nuclear family. Graham (1993) in her study of women caring for children in
Britain, suggests that it is preferable to

> 'adopt the term "families" as one used by many mothers to describe the
> domestic units in which they live and care for children' (Graham, 1993, p. 14).

How do boys learn to be men? It is often said, 'It's the women who bring up
boys', therefore it's women's fault if men are too 'macho'. But according to
Hite's research, the male respondents say that it is not women, even though
they have much greater contact in the early years, but men and other boys
who teach males their emotional identity. They complained that when they
were boys their fathers did not explain in any clear or positive way how to
be a man, but only criticised them for doing the wrong things, e.g. 'Stop
acting like a girl'.

Burgess and Ruxton (1996) suggest that the role of fathers (and other men)
became detached and deskilled as a result of the Industrial Revolution:

> For, over the last 150 years, fatherhood has been deskilled: mothers and
> others have taken on almost all the day-to-day functions which, when fathers
> worked at or near their homes, once bound fathers and children together.
> (Burgess and Ruxton, 1996, p. 5)

Sporadic efforts are being made to teach parenthood to boys and to
encourage fathers' involvement in their children's upbringing. In addition,

there are structural problems in the lack of rights for paternity leave and the employers' assumption that it is the mother's and not the father's responsibility to take time off for a sick child.

Gender socialisation starts at a very early age as the extract in Box 3.1 shows.

Box 3.1: Luke and Kezia

Luke and Kezia were twins, ten days old. We were to take them to the doctor for their ten day check. I dressed one in pink and the other in blue.

After the first few people we met I became aware of a clear difference in the way people related to each twin. Kezia was prodded in the chest, her head touched, patted even, or she was chucked under the chin. 'Who's a big little chap then?', 'You can see he's like his Dad', were the comments largely addressed to me. Luke, yes you're right, he was dressed in pink, was rarely touched but he was spoken to, 'Aren't you a beautiful little one then?'. There was eye contact made. Voices were softened. It sounded as if he was about half her weight although they were both the same. (Watts, 1995)

By the time they reach primary school, boys are negotiating their way through complex gendered relationships and negotiating hierarchies of friendship and alliances as the next two extracts show. It is taken from a study of six boys in one class in a primary school (Warren, 1996).

Box 3.2: Stephen

Stephen, in many ways, stands as an example of the dominant middle class masculinity within the school. He is highly competitive... He is also sporty... He shows a tendency for good intra-group skills and for working co-operatively with girls... (Warren, 1996, p. 212)

Boys who don't fit into the dominant norms have to adopt different survival strategies, as Andrew's story shows (Box 3.3).

Box 3.3: Andrew

Although Andrew is part of the high achievement group... He is seen by his parents as difficult and 'odd', and it is this oddness that Andrew appears to cultivate, particularly through his 'joker' strategy. (Warren, 1996, p. 215)

By adolescence the pressures of trying to develop an acceptable identity as a man can produce a huge sense of frustration which can lead to taking risks or to deviant behaviour as Peter's story shows (Box 3.4).

> **Box 3.4: Peter**
>
> I never was to find a way by which I could feel part of this new life (school)... Gradually, I withdrew... This unwillingness to allow teachers to reach me created the types of relationships and situations where I was seen to be at odds with the system, 'a disruptive influence' ... and by the time I'd reached fifteen I was desperate to escape and prove myself as a man, capable, independent and in control of my life... I blindly blundered off straight into the arms of the army. (Bruckenwell *et al.*, 1995, p. 26)

Masculinities

The most thorough up-to-date review of gender and masculinity is found in the recent book *Masculinities* by Connell (1995). In the first part of the book he examines psychoanalytic and social science perspectives on masculinity; the second part presents material from life history interviews with four groups of men; finally, the third part attempts to put masculinity in a global perspective, so that we don't just accept the Western experience as primary, and also examines the political implications.

Curiously, although the pressure to conform is so great, according to Hite (1994), most men do not feel that they are 'typically' male. Also most men do not feel that they are powerful. So many boys and men have to suppress their emotions in order to conform to something that deep down they don't feel comfortable with. Connell (1995) suggests that there are four perspectives on masculinities which explain how the dominant form of masculinity retains its power even if few men feel that they are part of the dominant group:

- *Hegemony*: the commonly accepted view that it is men who should hold the top positions in politics, military and police, and industry.
- *Subordination*: men who are gay are often oppressed, and 'coming out' is still risky for men in most sections of society. It may provoke violence, 'gay-bashing', or indirect discrimination.
- *Complicity*: many men do not meet the normative standards of masculinity but still go along with men's attitudes and behaviour towards women, ranging from sexist jokes in the workplace, through lack of involvement in parenting and housework, to direct physical and sexual violence towards women.

- *Marginalisation*: black and Asian boys and men meet direct racism on the playground and on the street and more subtle forms of discrimination at work and play. Black and Asian men are thus be forced to live and work 'on the margins'.

In Britain the dominant group is defined more specifically as white, middle-class, heterosexual, able-bodied men. The implications for men's health will be elucidated in Chapters 4, 5 and 6.

Connell (1995) shows that we need to examine 'conventional' masculinity from a historical perspective. The institutionalisation of warfare in the late nineteenth century has rationalised and legitimised violence for men against other men in the enemy countries and for protecting 'the women and children at home'. Fascism has been the clearest political exposition of the gendered state, but such ideas underlie all twentieth-century political statehood.

In industry, the shift from the masculine heavy industries to the 'information society' is still gendered: there is the assumption that it is boys rather than girls who have the skills and aptitude to work on computers in schools.

The concept and practice of team sports, which we nowadays accept as a key element of the construction of masculinity, has only become predominant since the beginning of the twentieth century. Men's bodies are hardened and used as weapons against each other, and the overcoming of injuries is seen as earning great respect. War and sport legitimise a public group form of male violence. Some would argue that this provides a necessary outlet and hence reduces private individualised violence on the street and in the home against women and children; others argue that the legitimisation of public violence encourages private violence.

In one sense these examples may offer us some hope: however solid seem to be the elements of masculinity at a particular time, these same elements can be unpacked and shown to have changed and be changing due to both conscious and unconscious developments (see Box 3.5 below). It is not, therefore, impossible that those elements which affect men's health can and will change.

Connell (1995) has added to the very limited stock of empirical studies of the dynamics of masculinities. He interviewed men in Australia whom he classified into four groups:

- *Live fast and die young*: working class men on the fringes of the labour market, who have experience of violent conflict with authority starting in school and subsequent involvement in petty crime, who have defined their masculinity *against* the hegemonic power structures.
- *A whole new world*: men 'who have attempted to reform their masculinity, in part because of feminist criticism', partly within the movement on environmental issues, who are trying to work on a non-gendered basis.

Box 3.5: Steve

I picked up the 'phone.

'Your Dad can't get off the commode', my Mum said shakily.

On their way to bed the previous evening Dad had fallen over, taking Mum with him. They had spent the night in chairs in the living room. Reluctantly I drove to Nuneaton. I'd been fighting the need to exchange roles with my parents and become responsible for them. As an only child in a house full of adults I'd felt responsible all my life – stopping my Nan leaving my Grandpa after another row. Later, guarding her as she gradually lost the power to reason. In my early 40s I made the commitment to be less responsible and more spontaneous.

Helping Dad from the commode to the settee took forty minutes; he veered between shouting in pain and anger and whimpering like a toddler, terrified of falling again. Later, as we all sat exhausted, he sighed deeply and when I asked him why he just said, 'I was thinking what a fool I've been'. I wish I'd asked him what he meant, but I couldn't.

I didn't want to be my Dad's carer; I took the role reluctantly. I found advocating for him difficult. Over the years we had drifted apart emotionally, to the point where we could hardly talk for more than a few brief phrases. I sometimes questioned if we had ever been close, but at his funeral I managed to remember seaside holidays, pitch and putt, long car journeys alone with him, fishing trips. I know we both wanted to be close, but something always got in the way. (Smith, 1998)

- *A very straight gay*: these are younger gay men connected with the flourishing gay community in Sydney. Unlike older gay men, they have little sense of the politics of the struggle in the 1970s and 1980s for public acceptance of homosexuality. They define themselves by an open gay identity but which is not effeminate and they do not reject friendships with women.
- *Men of reason*: these are men working in knowledge-based industries where technical rationality is a key element of their job. Their childhoods were mainly in conventional gendered families. They are aware of changes taking place in gender relations but find it difficult to accommodate easily to this in their personal lives with women.

What is striking about these abbreviated life histories is that, although Connell classifies them into four groups in order to illustrate his dimensions of masculinities, there is such diversity among all the men. Robertson and Williams (1997) have discussed how this view of masculinity as socially constructed is often in practice considered by health professionals to be less significant than biological essentialism and gender learning in infancy.

The challenge for this book is how we can carry out an analysis and develop a practice which recognises the diversity of masculinities and yet maintains a focus on the material and political factors which need to be understood in order to influence and change policy and practice.

National culture, masculinity and femininity

Hofstede (1980, 1991, 1998) has studied the influence of national culture on work goals in over 40 countries. One of the four (later extended to five) dimensions is masculinity–femininity (Mas/Fem) which he defines as follows:

> Masculinity stands for a society in which men are supposed to be assertive, tough, and focused on material success; women are supposed to be more modest, tender and concerned with the quality of life. The opposite pole, Femininity, stands for a society in which both men and women are supposed to be modest, tender and concerned with the quality of life (Hofstede, 1991, pp. 261–2).

Hofstede found that, although individuals can be both masculine and feminine at the same time, nations are predominantly one or the other and can be placed on the single Mas/Fem dimension. Although this research did not look specifically at health, subjective wellbeing was studied and shown to be related to the Mas/Fem dimension when national wealth was also taken into account. The potential for comparative research that links health to national culture, particularly the Mas/Fem dimension, looks promising.

Boys and masculinities

Having reviewed some of the views on the construction of gender and masculinity, we can examine how these concepts actually work in practice for different males and what can be done about them. Salisbury and Jackson (1996) have recently shown how the negotiation of their masculinity is a crucial part of growing up for adolescent boys. They offer practical ways of working in schools to challenge the most destructive patterns.

A much debated topic at present is boys' underachievement (Jackson, 1996). In the later 1970s the problem was seen to be girls' underachievement. Have things really changed for boys and girls since then or is it just that the focus of the academic and political debate has shifted? Jackson believes that many, perhaps most, boys have always underachieved at school but the problem of their lack of success was not considered important. Recent gender work in schools has been about empowering girls and not something that matters to boys.

The present destabilisation of . . . assumptions about boys in school is very contradictory. Either it can lead to a violent reassertion of heterosexual, macho culture . . . Or it can be seen positively as an historically unique moment to take action . . . changing boys' macho culture. (Jackson, 1996, p. 5)

Changing values

A survey of people's values in the age range 18–34 (Wilkinson, 1994) suggests that many younger women are now valuing autonomy, work and education more than family and parenting. These changes are partly driven by cultural change and partly by economic changes in the labour market. Some men are adapting and their values seem to be converging with women's, but about a third of these younger men, 'resisters', are failing to adapt. They still expect to be the breadwinner in heterosexual relationships even when traditional men's jobs are declining or nonexistent. They take much less involvement in domestic labour including parenting. For some men the only way to prop up their sense of masculinity is through involvement in drugs and crime. Currently this behaviour is being labelled 'social exclusion' by the Labour government (SEU, 1997). The survey shows that few older people have changed their values in the same way. However, the researchers consider that the changes in the younger age group are likely to be long lasting and will carry forward as they grow older.

The influence of the media on the formation of masculinity needs to be considered.

Despite the increase in so-called 'new men', the film and television industry still portrays masculinity as tough and violent, just wander round any video shop and you will see what I mean. I know that research into studies on violence is considered inconclusive – however, in the fifties children (particularly little boys) played 'Cowboys and Indians' *ad infinitum* no doubt due to the influence of Saturday morning westerns. In the seventies observation of children leaving school demonstrated that kung fu kicks were all the rage (Bruce Lee films?). Hollywood heroines no longer get tied to railway lines waiting to be rescued by the hero, or scream copiously at any hint of danger – but it would appear that the heroines of today echo the macho image of the hero, for example Kathleen Turner in *The War of the Roses* . . . the message being that if girls don't want to be victims they need to be tough as boys! My feeling about this stereotyping is that it is a great limitation on health education programmes, which have difficulty in competing with the more glamorous image of the movies. (Rose, 1999)

Perspectives on and analyses of gender

Since the analysis of gender, with emphasis on masculinities, is relatively new, it is necessary to be clear about the perspectives which are being adopted and the sources of the information. There are official government surveys, such as the General Household Survey (OPCS, annually), and regular national surveys such as British Social Attitudes (Jowell *et al.*, 1992). There are *ad hoc* surveys such as that reported in Wilkinson (1994). We have personal reports of men, although these are far fewer that are available for women.

Stillion (1995) has developed a multidimensional model which identifies the factors which influence early death among males. These are:

- *Genetic*: the XY chromosome which masculinises the fetus produces some of the risk of miscarriage.
- *Biological*: males produce increased levels of testosterone which is considered to contribute to aggressive behaviour and violence to others and to self including suicide and attempted suicide.
- *Developmental/cognitive/social*: as discussed above, the different socialisation of boys produces behaviour such as denial and repression of emotions and the taking of risks.
- *Environmental.*

Sexual attitudes and diversity

Sexual orientation

Diversity of sexual orientation may be universal in human societies but the levels of approval vary. In Britain, although heterosexuality has always been the norm, attitudes to homosexuality had been tolerant until the end of the nineteenth century, other than in the armed services. Homosexuality then became incorporated as a psychiatric disorder by the medical profession and it has only been decriminalised and demedicalised since the 1960s. Since the research of Kinsey *et al.* (1948), sexual orientation has begun to be recognised as a continuum which has important implications for sexual health and protection against HIV/AIDS.

A valuable source of information is the publication *Sexual Health Behaviour in Britain* (Wellings *et al.*, 1994) based on a national survey of sexual attitudes and lifestyles. One aspect of sexual behaviour that was not covered was 'the psychological and pleasurable nature of sexual relationships' (Wellings *et al.*, 1994, p. 7). This was the survey for which approval for government funding was suddenly withdrawn without explanation, although the *Sunday Times* speculated that it was Mrs Thatcher, Prime Minister at the time, who had personally vetoed the funding. The Wellcome Trust then provided the funds. The interviews were carried out between May 1990 and November 1991 and the final sample was 18 876.

Kinsey's seven point scale (Kinsey *et al.*, 1948) was reduced to a five point scale and two questions were asked about 'sexual attraction' and 'sexual experience'. Sexual experience was defined as:

> ... any kind of contact with another person that you felt was sexual (it could just be kissing or touching, or intercourse or any other form of sex). (Wellings *et al.*, 1994, p. 181)

The importance of this definition of sexual experience is that it is self-defined by the respondent and it is not defined solely in terms of sexual intercourse. The two questions are shown in Figure 3.1.

CARD K (M) (Q. 31a)
I have felt sexually attracted...

.... *only to females, never to males*	*(K)*
.... *more often to females, and at least once to a male*	*(C)*
.... *about equally often to females and to males*	*(F)*
.... *more often to males, and at least once to a female*	*(L)*
.... *only ever to males, never to females*	*(D)*
I have never felt sexually attracted to anyone at all	*(N)*

CARD L (M) (Q. 31b)
Sexual experience is any kind of contact with another person that you felt was sexual (it could be just kissing or touching, or intercourse, any other form of sex).

I have had some sexual experience

.... *only with females (or a female), never with a male*	*(R)*
.... *more often with females, and at least once with a male*	*(Q)*
.... *about equally often with females and with males*	*(T)*
.... *more often with males, and at least once with a female*	*(Q)*
.... *only with males (or a male), never with a female*	*(Z)*
I have never had any sexual experience with anyone at all	*(W)*

Figure 3.1 Sexual attraction for men to either sex. *Source: Wellings* et al. *(1994) p. 402.*

The results for men show that 93.3% and 92.3% report only heterosexual attraction and experience respectively; and 0.5% and 0.3% only homosexual attraction and experience respectively. There are thus 5% who report non-exclusive sexual attraction, and slightly less, 4.2%, who report non-exclusive sexual experience.

Sexual attitudes

One of the strengths of the survey is that it could look at how attitudes corresponded with reported behaviour. However, the relationships between attitudes and behaviour and the direction of causality cannot be taken for granted.

Only a minority of people were in favour of sexual intercourse being permitted for boys and girls before the age of 16 which is the legal age of consent.

Premarital sex is generally condoned whereas extramarital is generally disapproved of. There are only 8% of men and 10% of women who disapprove of sex before marriage, but more than three-quarters of men and even more women disapprove of sex outside marriage (Table 3.1). The biggest difference between men and women is in attitudes towards 'one night stands': whereas just over half the male respondents disapproved, more than 8 in 10 of the females disapproved. Men are less tolerant than women about same-sex relationships: more men than women disapprove of sex between two men and sex between two women.

Table 3.1   Views on sexual relationships.

	wrong or mostly wrong		
	men	women	difference
sex before marriage	8.2	10.8	2.6
sex outside marriage	78.7	84.3	5.6
one night stands	57.5	82.7	25.2
sex between two men	70.2	57.9	−12.3
sex between two women	64.5	58.8	−5.7

Source: Wellings et al. (1994) Table 6.5, pp. 246–7.

Views on homosexuality remain polarised: more than two-thirds of men and more than half of women believe that sex between two men is always or mostly wrong. Younger men and women are no more tolerant than older men and women.

Abortion is often considered to be a 'moral' issue, and continues to be strongly contested. On abortion the views of men and women are broadly similar. Women are *less* tolerant of abortion than men and younger people are slightly less tolerant than older people.

The researchers wanted to explore the hypothesis that there is consistency between people's views on a range of issues about sexuality. The answers to questions about the following eight topics were analysed by the principal components method which looks for common patterns of response:

- sex before marriage;
- sex outside marriage;
- sex outside cohabitation;
- sex outside regular partnership;
- one night stands;
- sex between two men;
- sex between two women;
- abortion.

The first principal component measures a scale of permissiveness associated with 'not wrong' answers to the eight questions. In general men are more permissive than women. For both men and women there is a strong age trend with older people being less permissive than young people.

The second principal component measures views of homosexuality. A majority of men are intolerant and a majority of women are tolerant. For both sexes there is not a strong age effect.

For these two components, permissiveness and homosexuality, the trend by age could be a 'true' age trend – as people grow older their attitudes change; or it could be a cohort trend – that society is becoming more tolerant and that this affects younger people more than older people and the younger people will carry the attitudes with them as they get older. A longitudinal study would be needed to investigate these two possibilities.

The state and patriarchy

The origins of the modern state in war and the raising of armies and then in control of violence through the police were essentially about men's roles in the public sphere. Part of the increasing involvement of the state in public health in Britain in the nineteenth century was in response to the poor health of recruits for the Boer War (Doyal, 1979) which led to the provision of school meals and school nurses carrying out health inspections.

Bryson (1992) provides a review of feminist critiques of the welfare state. She identifies the paradox that on the one hand many women look to the state for financial support and the provision of services other than in the family and reliance on a wage earning man, but also see that state as largely dominated by men and patriarchal views. In Britain, welfare thinking is still dependent on the views of Beveridge where welfare is built on the premise of the nuclear family.

This critique based on sex differences arose in the 1970s and had to struggle with the view of many intellectuals that only class-based analysis mattered. More recently there has been the criticism that the feminist critique assumed a white hegemony, and that an antiracist perspective on the welfare state exposes an inbuilt racism (Williams, 1989).

One of the key subjects of debate is 'the family'. It is not just a matter of sex differences, which was the main focus of the white feminist critique in the 1970s. For many black people 'families' offer protection against social and state racism, so that offers of help from health and social workers will be viewed with suspicion. People who are disabled feel that their needs for accommodation and the right to have children are not being met by class and able-bodied white critiques of the welfare state (Morris, 1991). Morris shows how political demands for abortion may be construed as 'eugenic cleansing' against disabilities.

The way in which the welfare state has developed varies greatly and Esping-Andersen (1990) shows that the British version does not fit in with the three more common models: liberal, corporatist, and social democrat. There is, therefore, a danger that an analysis of welfare and patriarchy in Britain should appear 'essentialist', and we need to take a comparative view and examine this relationship in some other countries. In Britain welfare is still seen largely as providing services in kind for the 'deserving poor'. The analysis of Le Grand (1982) has shown how since the Beveridge reforms after the Second World War it is the middle class who have received most benefit in many aspects of welfare.

Esping-Andersen (1990) shows that 'welfare' needs to be seen not solely in the sense of what we in Britain think of as the welfare services but also in terms of pensions and labour markets. As we shall be exploring the impact of social deprivation and economic poverty on men's health we need to set a basic structure for such consideration, and we hope that this book will form one step in a move towards developing a wider analysis of gender and health, and for moving towards gender-sensitive health policies and health services.

Sport

For boys in Britain sport is an apparently essential part of growing up and becoming masculine. The incorporation of team games in the late nineteenth century in Britain became part of the hegemony of masculinity, ironically at the stage when the British empire began its long decline. In one sense violence is legitimised. In health terms the benefits of physical exercise and the buzz of success at winning have to be balanced against the physical risks of sports injury and the psychological damage of failure. The professionalisation of sport and the importance of television and the large financial rewards of success need careful analysis. The recent professionalisation of rugby union with sudden involvement of millionaire business people and the increased exposure of television means that the bodies of professional sportsmen are subject to much increased wear-and-tear of the body as weapon (Sabo and Gordon, 1995)

Phillips (1984) has shown the important role that sport has taken, deliberately, in the formation of New Zealand as a nation. Referring to this, Connell (1995) comments:

> The device bridging the contradictions around masculine violence and social control was organized sport, especially rugby football... The exemplary status of sport as a test of masculinity, which we now take for granted, is in no sense natural. It was produced historically, and in this case we can see it produced deliberately as a political strategy. (Connell, 1995, p.30)

Disability

The social model

Oliver (1990) argues that people with impairments are disabled by the attitudes of able-bodied people. Official definitions of disability imply that the responsibility lies with the impaired individual whereas Oliver develops the social model of disability which places much of the responsibility in the structural features of capitalism and the organisation of the state and the associated attitudes in society. Definitions are important:

> Impairment – lacking part of or all of a limb, or having a defective limb, organism or mechanism of the body;

> Disability – the disadvantage or restriction of activity caused by a contemporary social organisation which takes no or little account of people who have physical impairments and thus excludes them for the mainstream of social activities. (Union of the Physically Impaired Against Segregation (UPIAS), 1976, quoted in Oliver, 1990, p.11)

The medicalisation of physical and mental disability is a feature of the late nineteenth and twentieth centuries. There has been more recently the emergence of organisations of disabled people at international, national and local levels. Although the disability movement has developed considerable lobbying power, nevertheless, the Disability Discrimination Act 1995 has been criticised for embodying the medical model.

There has been the tendency of assuming that 'the disabled' are homogeneous. Just like 'women' or 'men' there are people who are disabled with a huge range of impairments and diverse needs, and divided as much as united by class, ethnicity, age and gender.

Much of the more powerful writing about personal experience has come from women. Morris (1991) is a woman who became disabled through an accident. She has succeeded in writing a book which explains powerfully the personal experience of herself and other women, and links this to wider political and social trends. She finds links between the abortion debate and the eugenics movement and fascism and racism. Although the main emphasis of the book is from her feminist perspective, she does have a short section on masculinity and physical disability.

> The social definition of masculinity is inextricably bound up with a celebration of strength, of perfect bodies. At the same time, to be masculine is not to be vulnerable. (Morris, 1991, p. 93)

Gershick and Miller (1995) have explored the relationship of masculinity and physical disability by in-depth interviews with ten disabled men in the USA. They conclude that their sample of men adopt one of three main strategies: reliance, reformulation, or rejection.

Deafness

On looking into what seems to be a particular form of disability, we find considerable diversity. Deafness includes people who are born deaf and consider themselves to be part of the deaf community and for whom sign language may be their first language; people whose hearing becomes severely impaired *before* or *after* they have acquired speech, and whose abilities to speak and be understood, to hear, to lip read, to use hearing aids vary greatly; people who became deafened at work; people whose hearing becomes impaired as they grow older and who may, or may not, accept this as part of ageing.

People who consider themselves to be Deaf, that is part of the deaf community, have begun to develop expression of their culture through biographical and creative writing, in addition to the stronger political organisation and lobbying. Taylor and Bishop (1991) provide a collection of pieces about the experience of being deaf and becoming deaf.

Because of restrictions on the use of sign language until very recently, many deaf children were cut off from rich contact with many aspects of society (which we would expect to include information about health and sexuality).

> I remember feeling completely cut off from whatever was going on around me at school.... It was only through developing skill in BSL that I learned about the lives of the other children. But we were all at the same level! *Contact and conversation with adults to prepare me to face the world was totally lacking* [emphasis added]. (Clive Mason, in Taylor and Bishop, 1991, p. 86)

A deaf boy (or girl) in a mainstream school, intended to provide integration, may, in fact, have great trouble in learning about relationships.

> Nigel and his female equivalent Janie ... have a slight problem. They like girls/ boys, but they cannot work out what is going on between all the others. The

boys mutter in groups about 'wanking' and the best way to do it, whatever 'it' is . . . Nigel feels that he is not normal because he can't impress the girls and make them laugh . . . (Paddy Ladd, in Taylor and Bishop, 1991, p. 92)

Defining one's sexuality is bound to be influenced by disability as David Nyman explains.

I came out in October, 1978, after several years struggling with my own sexuality . . . I had considered myself as a bisexual for a while having had relationships with girls, but I had always wanted a relationship with a man. I suppose that the fear of being ostracised from the deaf community prevented me from doing that . . .

It is very difficult to be gay in the world of deaf people, as we do not conform to their standards . . . The deaf community is very small and many know each other; the deaf grapevine is a very powerful tool, and so we have to be very careful what we do. (David Nyman, in Taylor and Bishop, 1991, p. 173)

Andrew Charles is an African Caribbean deaf man who grew up in care. He comments on the influence of the segregation of the sexes in his school.

When I was first at school the boys and girls were kept separate. When I was older the school changed and the boys and girls were mixed for most school activities. I think that was better because when the sexes were segregated it led to a lot of homosexuality. I believe that is the reason why there are so many deaf-gay people now . . . By the time they left school their sexual preferences had been formed by their school experiences. (Andrew Charles, in Taylor and Bishop, 1991, p. 180)

Can men change?

The question, can men change, presupposes: (a) that 'men' form a homogeneous class, and we have been arguing strongly that we need to recognise diversity in men; (b) that men are not changing, and we have been arguing that gender is a dynamic process of development under change from politics, the media, local cultures, among other influences. We have also argued, as part of the paradox, that patriarchy is founded on a pervasive hegemony that strongly influences all men and women to some degree consistently.

From the point of view of men's health we can detect some changes that are progressive and some that are regressive. Whether individual men or groups of men can take conscious decisions and whether these decisions can influence wider networks and classes of men is worthy of debate. Connell (1995) has provided, as one of his four case studies of groups of men, examples of men attempting to reform their masculinity, which he calls 'a whole new world'. Segal (1997) has tried to provide an overview answer to the question and compares the situations in a number of Western industrialised countries. Part of her conclusion is that the answer must be closely linked to material conditions in capitalist economies:

> Such shifts as have occurred in gender roles in Sweden, however, remain severely limited by the continuing constraints of a capitalist economy and labour market which provide little scope for change in lifestyles, particularly for its sex-segregated manual workers. (Segal, 1997, p. 311)

The material conditions are supported by the individualistic ethos of competition and success at all costs closely bound into distinct gender roles.

Anti-sexist men

Christian (1994) has carried out one of the few empirical studies of 'antisexist' men in Britain, in contrast to the much larger literature in the USA, and furthermore of men living outside London. His book provides some interesting clues as to what motivates men to change and what are the necessary conditions for them to do so.

> My main finding was that more than three-quarters of the men had experienced a combination of two interacting and reinforcing influences in their lives: early life experiences which departed from conventional gender expectations; and adult experience of feminist influence, usually in a close relationship with an active feminist... (Christian, 1994, p. 183)

Among the features of their early life experience which appeared to have influenced their anti-sexist outlook were:

- non-identification with traditional fathers or identification with nurturing fathers;
- experience of strong mothers, usually involved in paid work;
- parents who did not conform to conventional domestic roles.

Some of these influences, particularly that of a close relationship with an active feminist, may have been relevant only to the particular cohort which Christian studied. With the lack of interest of younger women in being identified as a feminist (Wilkinson, 1994) this particular influence may have faded away although it may have been replaced by other challenges from women.

Christian (1994) makes a strong plea for more empirical research into the variations between heterosexual men.

> My view about much recent writing on masculinity is that often I cannot relate it to my own views or experience... In the context of hegemonic masculinity male sexuality seems to be socially constructed in terms of domination, but for

me sex is about shared pleasure not about dominating. Am I peculiar as a man in feeling this way? Or are there other unresearched non-predatory hetero-sexual men who feel as I do? (Christian, 1994, p. 188)

The answer to Christian's question in this quotation is that we don't know whether the majority of heterosexual men are predatory or not. The research has not been carried out. The national survey of sexual attitudes did not cover this issue.

Some men have had experience in anti-sexist men's groups but these groups have never cohered into an influential men's movement as some had hoped. For the men in Christian's sample being in a men's group was 'a phase in the lives of anti-sexist men, important but temporary' (Christian, 1994, p. 196).

Box 3.6: Jonk

Quite often when I come in after work I just collapse. Some men might come in and have a drink but we can't afford that . . .

With four kids, there is a lot to be done at home, and so really it is best not to stop and just get on. I find cooking much easier than Caroline does and so certainly when there is a tight time schedule, which there often is with the kids going to activities, it's best if I cook. I find if I get straight on with it that it's OK: as long as I don't stop I can manage to have the food on the table in time, and it's good food.

I have found that actually as long as I don't let myself stop I keep much more cheerful, though I do sometimes feel rather flat and that getting up in the morning isn't easy. I have found that my right knee is hurting quite often. I really suppose I ought to go to the doctor about it, but I really don't want to. I don't have the time and anyway what will he be able to do about it, it's probably just a sign of getting old. (Bruckenwell *et al.*, 1995, p. 39)

Younger men

What now seems to be happening with younger men, according to Wilkinson (1994), is a polarisation between men who have responded positively to changes in younger women's aspirations and those who are failing to adapt. Boys' underachievement in education is one of the features of this latter group. There is evidence of convergence in values between the 'progressive' younger women and men and which separates them increasingly from older women and men.

This divergence between the generations is an acute issue since so much of political and economic power resides with the older generation. The image of New Labour seems to be a conscious attempt to reach this generation. Whether the Labour government can meet their aspirations remains to be seen at the time of writing in mid-1998.

What is particularly important for our interest in diversity is how Wilkinson considers the debate is changing:

An older agenda of rights, that saw relations between men and women as a zero sum game, is being superseded by a much more complex set of issues: overwork for some and underwork for others; discrimination against men as well as women; sexual harassment by women as well as men; coping with the cultural barriers to male adaptation as well as the remaining barriers to women. (Wilkinson, 1994, p. 2)

The men's movement

Cooper (1990) has reviewed the 'men's movement' based upon limited documentary sources, mainly magazines, and interviews and his own participation. He considers that a movement never really existed, other than networks of very loosely linked temporary groups, and a few national conferences in the 1970s. Although men did consider that sexism and oppression of women should be challenged, very little of substance took place on these issues. Men have tried to liberate themselves from some of the constrictions of masculinity but this has not led to direct action to challenge sexism towards women.

It is possible the time scale which Cooper reviews is too short and the effects may be longer lasting but less direct than he is prepared to recognise. One argument is that direct action against the oppression of women is less important than men changing themselves and how they relate to women and children in their families and local networks. This argument certainly deserves to be debated. Just as 1970 feminists popularised the slogan 'the personal is political' men might reverse the slogan and say that 'the political should be personal'. Wider social attitudes need to be changed and the bottom-up approach is just as valid as the top-down approach.

There are some obvious parallels and lessons to be learnt for action on men's health. We have to ensure that a movement to improve men's health does not operate to consolidate men's power or to harm women's health. There should not have to be a zero sum game between the sexes.

Fathers

Compared with the empirical research and political debate about mothers there is a startling lack of debate and knowledge about fathers. Beyond the clichés we know very little. Since the work of Bowlby (1953) after the Second World War the emphasis has been on the essentialist biological role

Box 3.7: Dick

The Ten-Bob Note

Dad was a whizz-kid on his motorbike.
Knew his con-rods from his cam-shafts, like.

Mile-eating on the A Three-Six-Something
Spot of bother with the engine timing

Dad stops the bike, gets off, and has a look;
Teeth clenched. Grimaces. Spark plug's cooked!

Got to keep the bleeding ship afloat!
Dad swore, and fixed it with a ten-bob note.

Hated bricks, cement, but things metallic
Dad was master of. Smart-alec.

Wood, as far as he beheld it,
Couldn't be walloped, melted, forged or welded!

Had a son, very quick and bright
Mechanical, made Dad feel alright.

But then I come along, don't have the knack,
Dad said. Wallops me instead, gives me the sack.

They conned and shafted, **I** stayed in and cowed.
Two whizz-kids: company. Three, a crowd!

As a young boy I felt I had no place in the male world of my father, a world of mechanical ingenuity and skill with metal. At the age of two I developed asthma, which has remained with me ever since. Although it may be impossible to establish a causal connection between the illness and the feelings of rejection, it is worth considering in relation to the ideas about gender and emotional identity. (Leith, 1999)

of the mother. This has been disputed in feminist scholarship but debate on the actual or potential role of the father is notably absent. There has been more emphasis on the negative influence of fathers: the present father, whether through physical or sexual abuse; the absent father, whether actually living apart and not contributing practically or financially; or the father who works long hours and comes home after young children are asleep; the father whose only practical contribution is to take his son to the football match on Saturdays but does not offer any emotional support. We don't know how widespread are these negative images, and we don't have an equivalent archive of positive images.

There are, nevertheless, some positive examples which have shown that change towards more participative fathering is possible. A project in Australia (reported in Russell, 1983) showed success in fathers moving from traditional roles towards 'non-traditional shared care-giving'. The fathers reported how they had derived much more satisfaction from their interactions with their children.

In a small-scale project in Nottingham for fathers (Luczynski, 1996) it has been initially necessary to deal with the expressions of anger from the men. Some feel as if they have been kept out of the family by their partners, perhaps rightly so because of their lack of skills, and because their potential for violence may be seen to be dangerous towards their children. They may feel anger towards their own fathers which they have never got in touch with before. They may feel rejected by service professionals who are unused to working with men as in Alan's story, Box 3.8.

Box 3.8: Alan

When my children's mother and I divorced eight years ago, I became responsible for my two daughters through a bitter and hard process of negotiation and raw feelings. They ended up with me during the week, with their mother at weekends. A reversal of the usual settlement which made perfect sense in our case. I worked at home, their mother full-time in an office. I could switch my hours to suit school times, their mother couldn't. I could drop everything to be with them if they were sick.

Single mothers find support from each other easily; there is almost a social expectation that women alone with children will find company easily, will engender support as victims. But a single dad? Social rarities to most, they would not be seen as a group, nor supported as one. I have encountered surprise, bewilderment, admiration and ignorance. Never a feeling of support, of being as ordinary as a dad without his kids, or one still married.

I have had to grow, to feel and express feelings, because bringing up kids alone demands that. I have had to survive by juggling many tasks at once, because that is what running a home alone means. I have had to place their needs before mine only to find that I have gained too. (Taman, 1998)

Watts suggests that although there have been changes such as the presence of men at the birth of their children – this may nowadays be seen as a 'badge of manhood' – it is the more mundane aspects of family life and childcare which need to be illuminated.

Many men now attend the birth of their children. I think that most of us who have consider it an experience that we would hate to have missed. I have heard from many men, including those with very little awareness that it was the most important day of their lives. The number of us who find it thrilling to stand in the school playground, certainly at the 100th time, is substantially lower. Parenting is being there when the small child has grazed its knee; it's listening to the boring joke you've heard already ten times; it's getting up at 7 in the morning when they don't want to go to school . . . (Watts, 1997)

It is believed that Asian fathers of the 'third' generation who have grown up and been educated here are now taking a greater part in childcare and housework than their fathers or grandfathers did.

A recent review of fatherhood (Burgess, 1997) provides welcome historical and cross-cultural perspectives so that we can get away from the assumption that the current state of fatherhood in Britain is essential and unchangeable.

Men have been urged to keep at an emotional and physical distance from infants so that they will be cut off from their most tender feelings, so that they will be alienated from themselves. This has helped to condition them to blind obedience, has fitted them to undertake exhausting and degrading physical work, and has prepared them to be an army-in-waiting in times of peace, and to kill and be killed in times of war. (Burgess, 1997, p. 15)

Although it is very difficult to make any sound conclusions about historical changes in fatherhood, Burgess does suggest

That some fathers from all eras have been intimately involved in their children's upbringing is plain. And that, up to the middle of the nineteenth century, social structures made that involvement possible to an extent that seems unimaginable today is also clear. (Burgess, 1997, p. 71)

Although there has been a steady increase in awareness of the role of the father in childbirth and childcare, this has been mainly concentrated on middle-class white men in North America and Europe (Hewlett, 1992a). There is the danger that this develops into an ahistorical universalist assumption about fatherhood, for example, the ability to participate in childcare of many men who are employed is limited by long hours at work and time spent commuting to work.

Cross-cultural studies which would put western fatherhood into context are much more limited. Hewlett (1992b) has studied the Aka pygmies who are hunter-gatherers in central Africa.

Aka fathers provide more direct care and are near their infants more than fathers in any other human population that has been investigated (Hewlett, 1992b, p. 153).

This appears to be due to husbands and wives working together cooperatively in a variety of tasks both in the camp and when hunting. In addition, the Aka people have relatively abundant food supplies and are not involved in competition with other tribes, so that the men do not have to allocate large amounts of time to warfare.

Summary

In this chapter we have provided an overview of how boys and men are socialised to become masculine. This will form the basis for understanding behaviour in health and illness of men in Chapters 4, 5 and 6.

We started by distinguishing between biologically defined 'sex' and socially defined 'gender'. The first recognition of masculine identity by a baby starts in its family and, although most of the practical parenting is provided by the mother, the presence or absence of the father can be crucial to this development of identity.

Much of the diversity of masculinities can be explained by the intersection of gender with class, ethnicity and ability, although there are many gaps in our knowledge due to the scarcity of research and personal accounts.

The structure and resilience of masculinities rests on power relations. These are embedded in the state functions of violence, such as warfare, and control, such as policing; also in cultural practices such as sport where participants in contact sports such as football and rugby are encouraged to use their bodies as weapons; in work where the image of the heroic manual labourer is still a strong image even though there are very few such jobs left in Western countries. The current anxiety about boys' underachievement is partly explained by the lack of congruence between this work image and the opportunities which actually exist.

Sexuality is another important component of masculinities. Recent evidence shows that there is considerable fluidity in many men's sexual preferences and behaviour although this may not be recognised or socially accepted.

Finally in this chapter, we have attempted to answer the question 'Can men change?'. There is considerable evidence that younger women's attitudes are changing and that some younger men's attitudes are changing. However, a substantial proportion of men are being left behind by these changes, which is reflected in the boys' underachievement, and will be reflected in mortality and morbidity. In addition, our historical and cross-cultural review shows that many of the apparently rigid elements of masculinities have, in fact, changed or been changed deliberately in the late nineteenth and twentieth centuries. This offers hope that fundamental changes can take place in the future. Whether these changes will improve or reduce men's health has to be debated.

Further reading

Burgess, A. (1997) *Fatherhood Reclaimed. The making of the modern father*. Vermilion, London.
    Despite the vast literature about mothers, there has been little systematic study of fathers. This book provides a welcome introduction and the historical perspective helps to modify essentialist arguments and dispel prejudices.
Connell, R. (1995) *Masculinities*. Polity Press, Cambridge.
    This book provides an excellent review of psychological and sociological knowledge about masculinities; it contains four chapters of analysis of empirical data; and ends with a depth of analysis and projection which is outstanding.
Holland, J., Ramazanoglu, C., Sharpe, S. and Thomson, R. (1998) *The Male in the Head. Young people, heterosexuality and power*. Tufnell Press, London.
    A detailed empirical study of the construction of heterosexuality in young men and young women.
Salisbury J. and Jackson D. (1996) *Challenging Macho Values. Practical ways of working with adolescent boys*. Falmer Press, London.
    The importance of this book is that it provides a wealth of ideas for practical work with boys which comes from a critical analysis of theory and from wide experience.
Wellings, K., Field, J., Johnson, A. and Wadsworth, J. with Bradshaw, S. (1994) *Sexual Health Behaviour in Britain: the National Survey of Sexual Attitudes and Lifestyles*. Penguin, Harmondsworth.
    This is a readable account of the findings of a major national survey. It challenges many assumptions about rigid categories of sexual attitudes and behaviour.
Wilkinson, H. (1994) *No Turning Back: generations and the genderquake*. Demos, London.
    This book presents the results of a national survey of people aged between 18 and 34 which suggests major changes in values between generations and between women and men.

Chapter 4
Health and Illness Behaviour in Males

In this chapter we:

- present several frameworks or perspectives for analysing men's health;
- develop the argument that health is related to social capital and that relative poverty and the materialist explanation of the Black report are closely linked;
- describe how the suppression of emotion which is inherent in current masculinities produces overuse of alcohol, violence and mental distress;
- show that ethnicity is an important determinant of men's health, and that poverty within occupational class varies with ethnicity;
- describe the diversity of sexual behaviour which is related to attitudes to risk;
- show that individual 'lifestyle' behaviour varies far more than cross-sectional population surveys suggest.

Introduction

Our aim in this chapter is to apply the analysis of gender from Chapter 3 in order to understand men's health and illness behaviour which underlies the statistics of mortality, life expectancy and morbidity presented in Chapter 2.

There are a number of frameworks which we use including the 'dimensions of health' (Ewles and Simnett, 1992) and Dahlgren and Whitehead's (1991) model of the determinants of health. We also draw on the recent work of Wilkinson (1996) which relates health to social capital and which shows how relative poverty is more important a determinant of mortality than absolute poverty in industrialised nations. This is important for our analysis because men's access to social capital is qualitatively different, and often less robust, to that of women.

We examine men's suppression of their emotions and how this results in over-use of alcohol which is one way men deal with mental distress and

Real Men (Part 2)

Real men don't change their socks
Real men have big cocks

Real men lay bricks
Real men lay chicks

Real men don't mess up
Real men do press ups

Real men don't stutter
Real men fix their own gutters

Real men eat cow pie
Real men shave dry

Real men can take their drink
Real men don't need to think

Real men don't cry
And long before their time
They die

Dick Leith, 1998

This poem was based on the discussion of what it means to be a 'real man' at a meeting of South Warwickshire Men's Health Network.

which leads them into the criminal justice system rather than the mental health system. Recent research shows how ethnicity appears to be a determinant of mental ill health and of service response. The focus of the research has been black and Asian ethnic minorities, but the Irish also have particular needs which are often neglected because they are white.

Perspectives on health

The concept of 'health' needs to be disaggregated for the purpose of analysis, although the eventual intention is to aggregate or inter-relate these dimensions.

Dimensions of health

The dimensions of health adapted from Ewles and Simnett (1992) are:

- *Physical health*: concerned with the mechanistic functioning of the body.

- *Mental health*: the ability to think clearly and coherently – distinguished from emotional and social health, although there is a close association between the three.
- *Emotional (affective) health*: the ability to recognise emotions such as fear, joy, grief and anger and to express such emotions appropriately – also means of coping with stress, tension, depression and anxiety.
- *Social health*: the ability to make and maintain relationships with other people.
- *Spiritual health*: connected to religious beliefs and practices for some people; for others it is to do with personal creeds, principles of behaviour and ways of achieving peace of mind.
- *Societal health*: personal health is inextricably related to everything surrounding that person and it is impossible to be healthy in a sick society.

The social context for health

The model proposed by Dahlgren and Whitehead (1991) relates behavioural and social influences on health and is being widely used. It emphasises interactions between these different levels, for example, the way in which individual lifestyles are embedded in social and community networks and in living and working conditions, which are themselves related to the broader social, cultural and economic environment.

The Birmingham Public Health Report (Birmingham HA, 1995) uses the model to explain the different policy levels at which action can be taken to improve health and explores the role of the Health Authority at these levels. For example:

Level 1. Advocacy of broader health policies.
Level 2. Commitment to local health strategy in partnership with other agencies.
Level 3. Developing the capability of local communities and individuals.
Level 4. Screening for preventable risk factors.

Concepts of health

As well as the frameworks proposed by professionals and researchers it is important to understand what lay people mean when they talk of 'health' and how this influences their behaviour. Lay concepts of health have been researched since the 1970s by Herzlich (1973) and Blaxter (1990) among others. The main findings are that concepts of health have three main dimensions:

- health as absence of disease;
- health as the ability to cope with daily living and physical and mental stress;
- health as a positive state of well being.

But people cannot be expected to be completely consistent. A person may have contradictory views on their health at the same time.

These lay concepts of health have been explored in 'The Health and Lifestyle Survey' which was carried out in England, Wales and Scotland in 1984/5 (Blaxter, 1990). Since then there have been many regional and district lifestyle surveys but few, if any, have published such a thorough analysis and given such a deep discussion. These concepts have been analysed by sex and age but, surprisingly, not by ethnicity, and some key points are shown below.

The study examines in depth the relationship between social circumstances and health, which the Black report (Townsend and Davidson, 1982) called the 'materialist' explanation for inequalities in health, and found that this relationship changes by age and that the accumulated effects of disadvantaged lives were strongest in those in their 40s, 50s and 60s (Blaxter, 1990, p. 235):

- For young adults there were some differences but these were not great.
- In middle age the association was strongest, especially for men.
- Among older men and women health is more equal, perhaps because they are the survivors and the more disadvantaged have died.

Health inequalities and social capital

Wilkinson (1996) has shown that life expectancy has risen as countries develop economically (as measured by GDP) *up to a certain level*, but beyond that point further increase in life expectancy is related to the *decrease in income inequalities* and not to any further increase in GDP. He has related the increase in life expectancy to the change in relative poverty for 12 European countries from 1975 to 1985. Those countries with the greatest decrease in relative poverty show the greatest increase in life expectancy. The UK had the greatest increase in relative poverty in this period and the fourth lowest increase in life expectancy.

For England and Wales the life expectancy for women and men increased in every decade from 1901 to 1991, but by far the greatest increases in civil life expectancy (excluding military deaths) came in the two decades which included the First and Second World Wars. Both wars saw a return to full employment and a dramatic narrowing of income differences.

Social cohesion in a small town

The study of a small town, Roseto, Pennsylvania, USA, showed dramatic changes in life expectancy as social cohesion unravelled. The town had attracted attention because of the low death rates, particularly from heart attacks. This could not be explained by lifestyle factors such as diet, smoking and exercise. The population of migrant Italian-Americans had formed a close knit community with an egalitarian ethos. But as the community began to lose this cohesion in the 1960s the health advantage decreased:

> The data ... strongly suggests that the cultural characteristics... an emotionally supportive social environment is protective and that, by contrast, the absence of family and community support and the lack of well-defined role in society are risk factors. (Bruhn and Wolf, 1979, p.134, quoted in Wilkinson, 1996, p.118)

Mortality and gender in eastern Europe

Wilkinson (1966) did not single out gender in his study of health inequalities. However, the study of mortality and gender in eastern Europe (see Chapter 2, western and eastern Europe compared, p. 33) provides a 'natural experiment' (Watson, 1995) which shows the importance for health of people's subjective interpretations of objective conditions and how these differ between men and women. The data showed that between 1970 and 1990 male mortality rates had reduced for all western European countries and increased for all eastern European countries, whereas the pattern for women was not so distinct between western and eastern Europe.

Watson (1995) suggests that the changes were mainly due to the failure of state socialism to modernise in the 1970s and 1980s, before the liberalisation and overthrow of communism. People's expectations had been raised but no changes actually took place. So, although objective economic conditions had not changed, there was an increase in 'relative deprivation' because people's aspirations had increased. The gender difference was that women were, largely, able to gain some protection in the family,

> In line with Western findings, Polish research shows that women with paid work experience less stress than women who either have no family responsibilities or are not employed. (Watson, 1995, p.932)

For men, however, the traditional masculinity could not be released in the family and there was a tremendous lack of social activity that was not controlled by the state. In particular, for men who were not married, divorced or separated, death rates increased rapidly.

Social capital

Wilkinson (1996) relates national differences in mortality to the underlying social fabric which he describes as 'social capital' based on Putnam's definition:

> ...features of social organization, such as trust, norms, and networks, that can improve the efficiency of society by facilitating co-ordinated actions. (Putnam, 1993, p. 167)

Putnam carried out a longitudinal study of Italy covering a number of qualitative and quantitative measures which relate civic involvement, socio-economic development and institutional performance. Unfortunately, this unique study does not include health measures in institutional performance nor is civic involvement analysed by gender.

Wilkinson's (1996) main thesis is that an increase in income inequality reduces social capital which shows up in mortality rates. His data on national comparisons makes a convincing case.

Mustard (1996) discusses recent thinking about social capital and health, and summarises the efforts in the Canadian health sector at national and provincial level. He compares this with the much more fragmented efforts in the United States. When attention is given to building healthy social environments for children there is tension between rights of the individual and responsibilities of the community and state to intervene on behalf of children.

> There is understanding that building strong social capital will require some commitment of individuals to the needs of their communities and the changing social culture character of society. At present Canada has a more socially conscious society [than the USA] with a sense of the importance of social capital. (Mustard, 1996, p. 311)

This discussion of social capital identifies the need for national and intermediate levels of government and for communities to participate in building and maintaining social capital. This is a theme which we shall consider in Chapter 9. But the discussion does not take account of the gendered roles of men and women with respect to social capital nor does it consider the different needs of male and female children as they grow up.

Dealing with emotions

Emotions

> Emotional health: the ability to recognise emotions such as fear, joy, grief and anger and to express such emotions appropriately. (Ewles and Simnett, 1992)

Many men have difficulty in expressing their emotions. They have learnt to hide them because they are seen as an expression of weakness: see Box 4.1.

Box 4.1: Jonk

I hurt ... I hurt ... I hurt.

I find that I hurt difficult to admit. It hurts to say 'I hurt'. When I admit my hurt tears come to my eyes and my shoulder hurts even more. I'm embarrassed. I'm ashamed. I'm angry.

Don't be such a baby. Don't be wet. Who's shit scared?

I can hear all those voices. I can remember other times when I was hurt – and I learnt.

If someone shows they care, I fear. I fear that my camouflage has gone. I need to hide my hurt ... If they show me sympathy I might start crying – then I'll really be vulnerable. (Bruckenwell *et al.*, 1995, p. 22)

This seems to start very early as part of gender development. Much of the recent evidence about emotions is summarised in a recent popular book (Goleman, 1995). Although most of the material is North American, so that there has to be some care in assuming that it transfers directly to Britain, it does seem very plausible. He shows that parents tend to discuss emotions more with daughters than sons. Girls are more articulate in expressing their feelings in language whereas boys use physical expressions. Whether it is girls' facility with emotions which leads to their faster language development or the other way round is not clear. But there seems to be a synergy between language, emotions and play for girls which is not present for most boys.

> When girls play together, they do so in small intimate groups, with an emphasis on minimizing hostility and maximising co-operation, while boys' games are in larger groups, with an emphasis on competition. (Goleman, 1995, p. 131)

Some of the strategies for avoidance of expressing emotions are:

(1) valuing the rational over the emotional;
(2) the avoidance of intimate relationships;
(3) the use of addictive substances;
(4) intolerance of others expressing feelings.

(adapted from Meth and Pasick, 1996)

Some of the rules which men adopt for dealing with emotions which they see as acceptable are:

(1) Sports form an acceptable channel for expressing emotions, either as participant or spectator.
(2) Depending on women to fill their emotional needs.

(3) Using sex as an outlet for emotions.
(4) Assuming that alcohol or drugs permits and enhances expression of emotions.

(adapted from Meth and Pasick, 1996)

Suicide, risk taking and accidents

Suicide

Suicide has been given a great deal of attention since the publication of the Health of the Nation strategy (DOH, 1992), and two of the three targets for the key area of mental illness concern reductions in suicide rates. It is a particularly relevant topic in men's health because:

- suicides by men outnumber those by women by a ratio of more than 2:1;
- the suicide rate among young males aged 15–24 has increased by 75% since 1982.

Detailed information about the subject and its prevention is given in the review by the Health Advisory Service (HAS, 1995). Many of the risk factors are related to gender combined with mental ill health. Men living on their own as a result of being divorced or widowed have a higher risk. This suggests that these men who have lived with women have relied on them for emotional support and when the women die or leave the men cannot cope and resort to suicide.

There are factors related to employment and unemployment. The recent increase in suicides among farmers, perhaps associated with social isolation and ease of access to firearms, may be influenced by economic threats to their livelihood such as BSE. Unemployment or its consequences such as loss of possessions or status increases the risk of suicide. Because a man's identity is so dependent on his job and status in the world outside the family, if this goes the blow may be so severe that he will commit suicide.

For people who suffer mental illness high risk factors have been identified (HAS, 1995, p. 11):

- Depression – male, older
- Schizophrenia – male, younger, unemployed
- Alcohol addiction – male, age 40–60, disruption of relationships.

Mental distress, deviance and alcohol

Mental distress

Busfield (1996) proposes that mental distress has boundaries with physical illness, mental illness and social deviance. These boundaries are shifting, as a result of research findings and social change, and are contested as a result of struggles between different professional groups such as neurologists and psychiatrists. How a mentally distressed person expresses their distress and how they will be labelled and treated is strongly related to gender. For example, eating disorders have been recognised since the end of the nineteenth century as mainly a female phenomenon but it is only relatively recently that the conditions of anorexia nervosa and bulimia became formalised in medical terminology.

Patient statistics and community surveys show higher levels of depression in women than men. However it has been suggested that depression in men may be masked by alcohol and aggression:

> In Western culture men and women respond to psychological difficulties rather differently: women typically internalise their feelings and difficulties, becoming anxious and depressed; men turn them outwards either into excessive drinking or into aggression and violence. (Busfield, 1996, p. 93)

As Figure 4.1 suggests, more men than women may express their mental disorder in terms of social deviance and therefore be channelled into the criminal justice system, whereas women are more likely to be labelled as depressive and be treated in the mental health system.

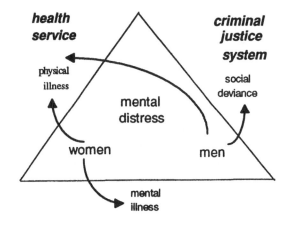

Figure 4.1 Gender and mental distress. *Adapted from Busfield (1996) p. 55.*

Men in the criminal justice system

Growing awareness in the criminal justice system (CJS) that there were considerable numbers of mentally disordered offenders has led to a growth in court diversion schemes. At the Victoria Law Courts in Birmingham the designated probation officer used to telephone the forensic psychiatric nursing service to ask for help and advice if they suspected a prisoner was suffering from mental illness. However it was felt that this was not fully effective. Therefore, a pilot study was set up (Sallah, 1992) involving the placement of a community psychiatric nurse (CPN) at the Law Courts:

- to assess the extent of mental illness among the population awaiting appearance in court;
- to advise the magistrates as to the best means of disposal.

During the pilot period, 27 February 1991 to 26 February 1992, 519 offenders were seen by the court diversion team. Of these, 290 (56%) were assessed as requiring mental health intervention (Table 4.1). The success rate is 77.5% of cases where psychiatric treatment is recommended by the CPN and accepted by the presiding magistrate.

Table 4.1 Recommendations to magistrates.

	Number	%
inpatient non-forensic	41	24.8
outpatient non-forensic	102	51.0
inpatient forensic	6	3.0
outpatient forensic	22	11.0
remand in CJS	29	14.5
total	200	100.0

Source: Sallah (1992), p. 72.

The ethnic origin of the population is shown in Table 4.2. This shows that African Caribbeans are over represented compared with the population where they form about 5% of the West Midlands population.

Before people reach the courts, when they are arrested and detained in the police cells, they may be suffering from some form of mental disorder.

Table 4.2 Ethnic origins of clients.

	number	%
white	361	69.6
African Caribbean	98	18.9
Asian	39	7.5
other	21	4.0
total	519	100.0

Source: Sallah (1992), p. 72.

Therefore a project was started in December 1992 which involved the placement of a CPN at a police station in Birmingham to screen people who are arrested for any mental illness.

A recent report on the Birmingham Court diversion scheme for January–June 1998 shows statistics which are very similar to those for 1992 in Tables 4.1 and 4.2 for recommendations to magistrates and for ethnicity of those assessed (Hillis, 1998).

Health of men in minority ethnic groups

The Fourth Policy Studies Institute survey

The Fourth National Survey covered a large nationally representative sample of 5,196 people of the main minority ethnic groups in Britain, together with a comparison sample of 2,867 whites (Nazroo, 1997a).

Because of the effects of differential migration it is necessary to standardise the data by age and gender. In most analyses and cross-tabulations Indians and African Asians (I&AA) are combined and Pakistani and Bangladeshi (P&B) are combined. However, there are situations where there are significant differences between the groups which have been combined.

Respondents were asked to provide a global self-assessment of their health over the preceding 12 months compared with people of the same age, see Table 4.3. The proportion of men who reported their health as fair, poor or very poor, was 26% of the white sample (Nazroo, 1997a, Table 2.2, p. 18). The proportions for the minority ethnic groups were:

- *Pakistani* (34%) and *Bangladeshi* (35%) men were much more likely to describe their health as fair or poor compared with whites.
- *Caribbean* men (33%) more likely to describe their health as fair or poor compared to whites.
- *Indian* and *African Asian* (26%) were similar to whites.
- *Chinese* (20%) were less likely to describe their health as fair or poor compared to whites.

For all ethnic groups including whites, the proportion of men was lower than women by 4–6%, except for African Asians where the proportion of men was only 1% less than women.

Overview of health findings

When comparing minority ethnic groups, the following trends emerged:

- Pakistanis and Bangladeshis were particularly disadvantaged on the general health assessment and coronary heart disease.

Table 4.3   Self-assessment of health.

	Report of health compared to others of same age	
	men with fair/poor health	women with fair/poor health
all ethnic minorities	29	35
Caribbean	33	39
all south Asians	29	33
Indian	26	32
African Asian	26	27
Pakistani	34	38
Bangladeshi	35	41
Chinese	20	28
white	26	32

Source: Nazroo (1997a), Table 2.2, p. 19.

- Caribbeans were worse on the general health assessment and for respiratory symptoms and hypertension.
- Indians, African Asians and Chinese reported general health and particular conditions quite similar to whites.
- Respiratory disease – ethnic minorities reported less prevalence than whites (differences were mainly due to patterns of smoking).

There may be several different explanations for these findings.

- *Artefactual*: questions may be interpreted differently by different ethnic groups.
- *Effects of migration*: age distribution of migrant and non-migrant ethnic minority populations in Britain are very different.
- *Racial harassment*: although the experience of racial harassment may be related to health, it cannot explain the pattern of ethnic variations in health reported here.
- *Socio-economic effects*: when households divided into non-manual, manual, no full-time worker, there is a clear effect of class on self-reported health, see Figure 4.2.

Variations within socio-economic bands

The variations obtained emphasise the importance of investigating social class in more depth. The mean income within class varies by ethnic groups, Table 4.4. For each class the mean income for the minority groups is less than for whites, and for Pakistanis and Bangladeshis is much worse.

The mean duration of unemployment for whites is seven months, whereas it is 12 months for Indians and African Asians, 21 months for

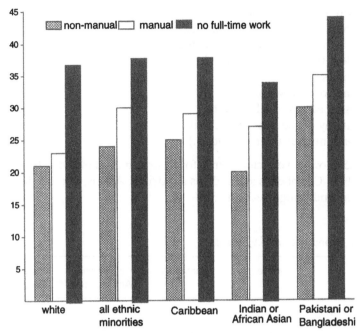

Figure 4.2 Health reported fair or poor by class and ethnicity. *Source: Nazroo (1997a), Table D.1, p. 204.*

Table 4.4 Income by class and ethnicity.

	white	Caribbean	Indian and African Asian	Pakistani and Bangladeshi
mean income by Registrar General's class (£)				
I/II	250	210	210	125
IIIn	185	145	135	95
IIIm	160	145	120	70
IV/V	130	120	110	65
percent lacking one or more basic housing amenities				
owner occupiers	11	12	14	38
renters	27	23	28	37

Source: Nazroo (1997a), Table 5.2, p. 99.

Caribbeans and 24 months for Pakistanis and Bangladeshis (Nazroo, 1997a, Table 5.2, p. 99).

Another approach to measuring disadvantage is to develop indicators of standard of living. Nazroo (1997a) uses:

Poor, with any of the following:
- overcrowded accommodation;
- lacking sole access to amenities;
- less than four consumer durables.

Good, consists of all:
- not overcrowded;
- sole access to all amenities;
- many of the consumer durables.

(*Medium* is neither Poor nor Good.)

Table 4.5 shows a very clear curve for *Poor* standard of living from 8% of whites, 14% Caribbeans and Indians & African Asians, to much higher for Pakistanis and Bangladeshis at 50%.

Table 4.5 Standard of living by ethnicity.

	white	Caribbean	Indian and African Asian	Pakistani and Bangladeshi
Standard of living				
Good	43	23	34	9
Medium	49	63	52	41
Poor	8	14	14	50

Source: Nazroo (1997a), Table 5.3, p. 101.

These findings indicate a clear hypothesis that the relatively deprived socio-economic positions of ethnic minority groups compared with whites contributes to their poorer health.

Men's reaction to illness

So far we have been discussing men and their attitudes to and behaviour about health. In this section we consider how men react when they become ill. We shall see how gender affects how men react when they first recognise symptoms and whether they seek help; and we shall see how men react when they have been diagnosed and brought into the health service. In Box 4.2 David describes his reactions to the operation to have his pacemaker renewed and how it brings out suppressed memories from his childhood.

In Box 4.3 Jim describes the initial reactions to symptoms of a hernia and how he tried to avoid taking action and getting advice. He does not want to worry his doctor.

Box 4.2: David

I'm lying on my back, spreadeagled beneath the camera while it's sending images of my heart and pacing wire to the technicians at the back of the theatre. It's difficult to keep a whole sense of who I am in that tethered position. I feel like a trapped pig in a slaughterhouse...

Conflicting voices from my childhood begin to wrangle inside me again. The 'grin and bear it' voice is arguing for grim stoicism and heroic control as a 'real man'. But my other voice – of a very frightened helpless boy – is trembling and shaky... Twisted up, bully boy faces from my secondary school are peering down at me. Fatty Rowe with a broken nose and vicious piggy eyes. Tubby Heath – oily, smirking, barbed. (Jackson, 1997)

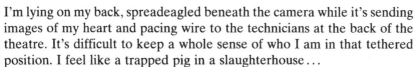

Box 4.3: Jim

I think I have one. I don't remember getting it, not like a cut finger or a sprained ankle. You know exactly what happened and how it happened.

Over two, maybe even three, years ago I was aware of a sharp pain like a burning sensation in my right groin. It didn't happen very often and only came on when I had been walking a long distance or standing about all day which wasn't very often and anyway the pain always stopped after a short rest... How could it be a hernia? I had two full medical checkups from my GP since the pain started, he was always into annual checkups, even before they became popular: the full works, strip to your underpants, touch your toes, lower the pants, hand on the groin, 'cough'. Well he never found anything wrong so how could it be a hernia? I suppose I should have mentioned it, but it seemed so trivial and after all doctors are very busy people and you don't want to worry them with little things like a suspected hernia. If I had one he would have found it, wouldn't he? (Source: Bruckenwell *et al.*, 1995, p. 23)

In Box 4.4 Chris describes how he had to come to terms with the first serious illness in his life, a testicular tumour.

Male cancers

Testicular cancer

When a cancer occurs it is usually on only one of the testes. The testis develops a lump, which feels harder or less smooth. The results of treatment are very good provided that it is treated early. Cancer of the testis is relatively uncommon in the whole male age range but is most common in the

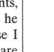

Box 4.4: Chris

I first began to get an occasional pain in the top of one testicle. I also noticed that the surface of the testicle was a little bit rough... I waited for it to go away. It didn't. I hate doctors' surgeries at the best of times – and it was a long time since I had been to see my GP, I didn't even know if she was still there. It was also difficult to take a morning off work or leave early one evening in order to get an appointment.

[after the ultrasound diagnosis] I never imagined that I would become a helpless and uninformed victim of the health service regime. I wanted to ask what it was, how bad it was, what they would do with me, but instead I took these worries away with me.

[after the operation to remove the testicle with the tumour and follow-up radiotherapy] I am aware how fragile health is, and can no longer hide behind the assumption that it is always someone else, never me. I have plans to become fitter and healthier than before, to keep work in perspective and to take more care of my needs. (Ryan, 1995, p. 56)

20–34 age range. The UK incidence has been increasing in the 1990s, as in many other industrialised countries, but there is no agreed cause. However, the death rate has been decreasing because early diagnosis is improving and treatment is getting better. The incidence and mortality for the 15 health districts in the West Midlands Region in 1995 showed no relationship to poverty measured by Townsend score (NHSE-WM, 1995). There is, however, a higher prevalence in the wealthier districts because people live longer there, Figure 4.3.

Prostate cancer

Prostate mostly affects older men. Prostate cancer varies greatly between different countries. Although the measured incidence is increasing this is partly due to ageing populations and partly due to improved awareness and diagnosis. There is, however, considerable debate about the safety and effectiveness of both diagnosis and treatment procedures. The incidence and mortality for the 15 health districts in the West Midlands region in 1995 showed a slightly higher rate in the wealthier districts measured by Townsend score (Figure 4.3).

Michael Korda (1997) has written a book about his experience of prostate cancer in which he explains the problems he had and other men have in facing up to the risks and why they ignore signs and seeking help:

> ... prostate cancer is the biggest fear of most men. It carries with it not only the fear of dying, like all cancer, but fears that go to the very core of mascu-

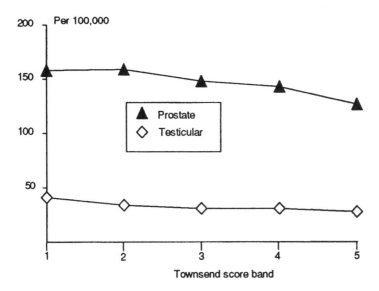

Figure 4.3 Prevalence of testicular and prostate cancer by Townsend score. Adapted from NHSE-WM 1995. *Data source: West Midlands Cancer Intelligence Unit.*

linity – for the treatment of prostate cancer, whatever form it takes, almost invariably carries with it well-known risks of incontinence and impotence that strike directly at any man's self-image, pride, and enjoyment, and which, by their very nature, tend to make men reticent on the subject. (Korda, 1997, pp. 3–4)

Michael Korda is a senior executive in a well known US publishing company so his feelings and his experience of treatment, with his ability to write about it, may be different from that of many British men and men who work in low level jobs or are unemployed. He suggests that many men, on being told that they have prostate cancer, are initially more worried that they are going to lose their job than that they are going to die. In the USA the loss of a job can mean loss of health insurance which does not apply in countries with universal health services.

The lack of knowledge about male cancers appears to be extensive in Britain as a recent survey has shown (MORI/ICR, 1998). The level of awareness in 1998 of testicular and prostate cancer had increased by about 5% since a similar survey in 1995, but is still low. This compares with men's greater knowledge of other health problems including heart disease, lung cancer and even of breast cancer. 80% of men had never heard of the blood test for prostate cancer (PSA). A significant proportion of men said that they would not undergo surgery if there was a risk of incontinence or impotence.

Ethnicity and mental health

This was a part of the Fourth National Survey of Ethnic Minorities conducted by the Policy Studies Institute (PSI) in partnership with Social and Community Planning Research (SCPR) (Nazroo, 1997b). The survey included a matched sample of white respondents which itself included subsamples of people with Irish family origins and other whites with neither Irish nor British family origins.

Mental illness

The classification of mental illness used in the survey consisted of:

- *psychosis*: which 'typically involves a fundamental disruption of thought processes...';
- *neurosis*: separated into anxiety and depression.

Psychosis

Previous research has shown much higher rates of psychosis among African Caribbeans than whites and other minority ethnic groups. However, much of this research is based on hospital admission rates and not on community surveys. There has been considerable disagreement about possible explanations. Factors suggested include: consequences of migration; differences in biological or cultural factors; discrimination and racism that people from minority ethnic groups face in Britain; flaws in the way in which the data are collected and analysed.

Data from this community survey show different results: Table 4.6. Here we see that for males by far the highest prevalence rate per thousand is for Irish and other whites, more than twice that for white; the rate for Carib-

Table 4.6 Prevalence of non-affective psychosis by ethnicity.

	white	Irish or other white	Caribbean	Indian or African/ Asian	Pakistani	Bangladeshi	Chinese
			rate per thousand				
Gender–age standardised							
Male	8	21	10	6	5	5	3
Female	8	7	17	6	6	4	0

Source: Nazroo (1997b), Table 3.6, p. 41.

bean men is only slightly greater than for white men; men in the three South Asian groups and the Chinese have much lower rates. For whites and South Asians the rates are very similar for men and women. However, for Irish and other whites the rate per thousand for men, 21, is much higher than for women, 7; whereas, for Caribbean the position is reversed with the rate for women, 17, being higher than for men, 10.

Neurosis

The prevalence of neurosis–anxiety is shown in Table 4.7. The rates for male and female Irish and other whites are both much higher than for the same gender in all the other ethnic groups. For all groups female rates are higher than male rates, although the difference for Pakistanis is small.

Table 4.7 Prevalence of neurotic anxiety by ethnicity.

	white	Irish or other white	Caribbean	Indian or African/ Asian	Pakistani	Bangladeshi	Chinese
cell percentages							
Gender–age standardised							
Male	12	23	11	8	10	2	5
Female	23	32	14	11	11	7	10

Source: Nazroo (1997b), Table 3.3, p. 38.

The prevalence for neurosis–depression is shown in Table 4.8. Here the rates for Irish and other whites and Caribbean are similar for each gender and higher than the other groups. For all groups except Pakistani the rate for females is higher than for males.

Table 4.8 Prevalence of neurotic depression by ethnicity.

	white	Irish or other white	Caribbean	Indian or African/ Asian	Pakistani	Bangladeshi	Chinese
cell percentages							
Gender–age standardised							
Male	2.7	5.8	5.6	2.5	3.8	1.6	1.6
Female	4.8	6.8	6.4	3.2	2.9	2.2	1.7

Source: Nazroo (1997b), Table 3.3, p. 38.

Key findings

Prevalence of psychosis within Caribbeans was somewhat higher than for whites, but nowhere near the difference shown in treatment statistics. The difference was due to Caribbean women not to men. There was no evidence of an age effect, nor was there a difference between migrants and non-migrants.

Sociodemographic factors are important influences on mental health, perhaps greater than ethnicity, but the direction of causality is not always clear.

There is a growing body of evidence that suggests that Caribbean patients are more likely to be treated coercively. Quality of care may be related to ethnicity, communication with health professionals, and to geographic location in inner city areas with poor quality primary care facilities.

The mental health of Irish men

Data from the PSI survey (Nazroo, 1997b) shows that Irish men have higher rates of psychosis, Table 4.6, neurotic anxiety, Table 4.7, and neurotic depression, Table 4.8., than whites and all other minority ethnic groups. Bracken *et al.* (1998) provide a short review of the lack of knowledge about these issues and recommend:

> ...the continued neglect of this community in Britain is now untenable. In particular, there is an urgent need for both quantitative and qualitative research relating to the mental health needs of Irish immigrants. (Bracken *et al.*, 1998, p. 103)

Sexual behaviour

There has been considerable research on 'lifestyle' factors such as diet, smoking, alcohol consumption and exercise, but surprisingly little on sexual behaviour, and on the possible relationships between physical health and sexual behaviour. In the National Survey of Sexual Attitudes and Lifestyles (Wellings *et al.*, 1994) questions were asked about perceived health, chronic illness, alcohol consumption, smoking, height and weight in the face-to-face interview.

For self-reported health status across both sexes and all age groups well over half the respondents reported their health as 'very good' or 'good'; with the proportion reporting 'poor' or 'very poor' increasing slightly with age. Analysis by marital status showed little difference for 'very good' or 'good' between the categories married, cohabiting, widowed, divorced or separated, and single for men and women. Widowed men, however, reported 'poor' or 'very poor' health more frequently than widowed women; and both divorced or separated men and women reported higher levels of 'poor' or 'very poor' health than those in other categories of marital status.

There was only a weak relationship between perceived health and heterosexual intercourse. This was mainly because those who experienced no intercourse within the last four weeks more frequently reported poor health.

There was a strong relationship between smoking and number of heterosexual partners in the preceding year, Figure 4.4. This applied to men and women, and across age groups and across the marital status groups.

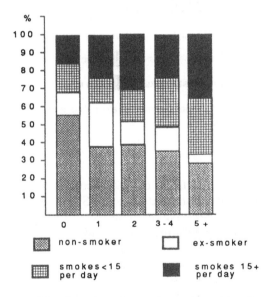

Figure 4.4 Number of female partners for men by smoking status. *Source: Johnson* et al. *(1994), Table A5.4A, p. 452.*

The relationship between alcohol consumption and number of sexual partners might be expected to show a similar relationship to smoking for the circumstances in which it is consumed and the lessening of inhibitions may stimulate sexual activity and finding a new partner. The survey did show such a result for both men and women: Figure 4.5.

There are, therefore, links between a number of risk-taking behaviours. For smoking the relationship was stronger for men than women, whereas for alcohol consumption the relationship was stronger for women than men.

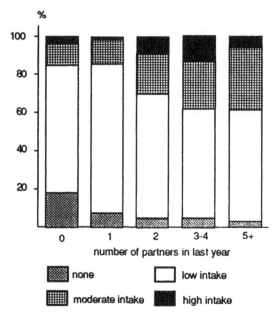

Figure 4.5   Number of female partners for men by alcohol consumption. *Source: Johnson* et al. *(1994), Table A5.4A, p. 452.*

Risk reduction

The most obvious adverse effects of risky sexual activity are unplanned pregnancy and sexually transmitted diseases (STD) including HIV/AIDS. The most common contraceptive methods used in heterosexual sex were: the pill (29% women and 30% men), the condom (26% women and 37% men), and sterilisation (23% women and 21% men). The trend towards more male than female sterilisation has grown in recent decades. Male sterilisation is less frequent in social classes IV and V.

There has been some exploration of how contraceptive use varies for women during their life and also the generation effects, for example the introduction of the pill followed by the discovery of side-effects. There has not, however, been any similar degree of study of men's pattern of sexual behaviour and use of contraceptives.

Safer sex

An openended question was asked in order to find out how people interpret safer sex:

There has been a lot of publicity about AIDS in the last year or two. From what you have heard or read, what does the phrase 'safer sex' mean to you?

By far the most frequent response was 'use of condom' (men 75% and women 81%); the next most frequent responses were 'monogamy' and 'restrict number of partners' (around 30% for men and women).

The prevalence of unsafe sex (two or more heterosexual partners and no condom use in the last year) was highest in the 16–24 age group (men 9.7% and women 9.2%) (Table 4.9). It showed considerable difference between the marital status groups, with widowed/divorced/separated men highest. This may be a group who is not easy to reach with conventional health education interventions.

Table 4.9   Unsafe sex by age and by marital status.

	men %	women %
age group		
16–24	9.7	9.2
25–34	5.8	3.8
35–44	5.7	3.1
45–59	3.7	1.6
marital status		
married	3.0	1.3
cohabiting	10.4	5.7
widowed/separated/divorced	15.7	8.0
single	9.6	10.6

Source: Wellings et al. (1994), Table 8.10, p. 363.

Health and lifestyle

Lifestyle in health policy

People bring their 'existing health' to work. Their health could have been affected positively or negatively by their lifestyle, and is a reflection of individuals' values, beliefs, priorities and interactions with health systems. Lifestyle is a difficult term to explain, people have a notion of what it means, but it will mean different things to different people. In the past, lifestyle was seen as something which was purely the responsibility of the individual, a responsibility in which the state and society had a minimal part to play.

> To a large extent though, it is clear that the weight of responsibility for his own state of health lies on the shoulders of the individual himself. (DOH, 1976, p. 38)

This view has changed, and the publication most responsible for this change was the Black report (Townsend and Davidson, 1982). The report was not well received by the government of the day when it was presented in 1980, and there was a strong move to discount the major recommendations and the general thrust of the arguments that inequalities in society lead in some measure to inequalities in health. The variations in health and disease could not be discounted just on the basis of behaviour of individuals. Other social factors such as income, education, occupation, housing and diet also needed to be considered when looking at a person's health.

The view of a more rounded and wider embracing approach to looking at health and lifestyle was emphasised by the Health For All by the Year 2000 activities following the WHO Alma Ata declaration in 1978:

> The main social target of WHO in the coming decades should be the attainment by all citizens of the world by the year 2000 of a level of health that will permit them to lead a socially and economically productive life. (WHO, 1985, p. 1)

The European Region of WHO issued 38 targets for Health For All in 1984 (WHO, 1985). Targets 13 to 17 relate to lifestyle and include areas of concern such as healthy public policy, social support systems, knowledge and motivation for health behaviour, positive health behaviour, and health damaging behaviour. This acknowledges the need for public policy and social intervention as well as individual responsibility. A report from an independent multidisciplinary committee, *The Nation's Health* (Smith and Jacobson, 1988), looked at the health of the nation, that is, both the current patterns of disease and of health-related behaviour.

The report, which is very comprehensive and unusually incorporates health in the workplace, continues to develop the theme of shared responsibility for health. The report, by focusing on disease and health behaviour, addresses many lifestyle issues: circulatory disease, cancers, alcohol, AIDS, road safety, tobacco, diet, sexuality and reproductive health. From this wealth of information the final part of the report identifies a strategy for public health interventions which would have significant health benefits. The main areas of concern are not too different from the European Regions targets for Health For All. This is to be expected, but the supporting evidence links the problem areas with areas of professional and political interaction.

The emerging or re-emerging of a stronger public health approach to health is evident in the late 1980s (WHO, 1985; Smith and Jacobson, 1988; Ashton and Seymour, 1988). The current focus is moving back towards the earlier health philosophies of the late 1800s and early 1900s that the emphasis must be on prevention, and on a corporate, community basis rather than expecting individuals to take total responsibility for their own health and to control factors beyond their capacity to do so. The move now is towards 'healthy cities', seeing individuals, families and government within a social and cultural setting in which everyone has a role and part to play in maintaining a healthy lifestyle and therefore contributing to the health of the nation (Ashton and Seymour, 1988). This development has resulted from the obvious failure of 'health systems' to improve the health of the nation beyond a certain point. There has been a revisiting of public health issues, a greater awareness of the individual, the family and the community in relation to health care; a greater acknowledgement of the need to empower people to take responsibility for their health in partnership with others.

The emergence of the 'green' movement may have been a prime force for this development. Disasters such as Bhopal and Chernobyl have caused incalculable ecological and environmental devastation. There is increased social awareness of the diminishing resources of the world and the fragility of the current infrastructure in protecting those resources.

Blaxter (1990) continues the research into lifestyle and health, and acknowledges the wide ranging and multifactorial nature of the term. The White Paper *The Health of the Nation* (DOH, 1992), was intended to be a cross-departmental publication suggesting a framework for a strategy for health, focusing on key target areas, with suggested targets for success. Further reference will be made to this and other publications in the analysis of results from this survey.

The debate about lifestyle explanations

The Black report (Townsend and Davidson, 1982) proposed four theoretical explanations for the relationship between health and inequality:

- artefact;
- selection;
- materialist;
- behavioural.

They favoured the materialist explanation although recognising that at that time suitable information was not available. They commented on the behavioural explanation:

> Such explanations ... often focus on the individual as a unit of analysis emphasizing unthinking, reckless or irresponsible behaviour or incautious life-style ... (Townsend and Davidson, 1982, p. 110)

The Conservative government, who had come into power while the Black report was being developed, rejected the materialist explanation and, subsequently, put emphasis on the behavioural explanation. A review of the Black report ten years later felt that research had been biased, and probably funded, towards the behavioural at the expense of the materialist.

> Most importantly, the neglect of the area that the Black report described as materialist should not continue. Unfortunately, the studies of the social distribution of health currently being conducted seem to be focused on the much investigated topics of lifestyle and selection. (Davey Smith *et al.*, 1990, p. 376)

It is only in the past few years that research on the materialist explanation is beginning to come to fruition (Wilkinson, 1996 and 1997).

Despite the above criticisms, lifestyle surveys do provide valuable *descriptive* information which should not be confused with causal explanation. There have been national surveys such as the Health and Lifestyle Survey described below, and many regional health authorities and district health authorities have carried out lifestyle surveys. At the least these surveys do provide snapshots of health behaviour.

The Health and Lifestyle Survey

The first Health and Lifestyle Survey (HALS1) was carried out in 1984/85 with 9003 respondents (Blaxter, 1990). A second longitudinal survey (HALS2) was carried out in 1991/92 which followed up the original respondents, and achieved 5352 completed contacts. It is, therefore, particularly valuable because there have been so few longitudinal surveys (Cox *et al.*, 1993).

Demography

One of the valuable pieces of evidence from a longitudinal survey is to show that demographic changes are taking place. These do not show up in a repeated cross-sectional survey which, therefore, gives an unrealistic static impression of people's lives. Although the overall household structure does not change in proportional terms, many people have moved from one category to another. For men in the 39–59 age group at the time of the HALS1 survey who were living as a couple with dependent children, only 32% were still in this household category at the time of the HALS2 survey seven years later, 50% were living as a couple with adult children, and 13% as a couple without children. The above changes in household structure form part of life changes such as forming partnerships, having children, dissolving partnerships.

Changes in socio-economic groups are also an important part of the dynamics of society which do not show up in cross-sectional statistics. For males in the younger age group 18–38 at the time of HALS1 considerable changes took place up and down the scale. Some of these changes would be due to students and unemployed being classified by a parent's socio-economic grade (SEG) at HALS1 and by their own employment at HALS2. It is probable that non-respondents may have been more mobile and more changeable than respondents. Of men aged 18–38 who were unemployed at HALS1 60% were employed at HALS2, although the overall rates of unemployment were similar in the two surveys: Figure 4.6.

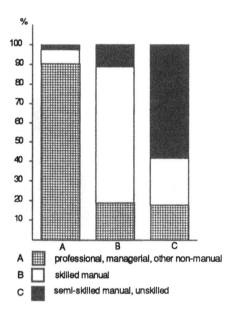

Figure 4.6 Changes in socio-economic grade between HALS1 and HALS2 for men aged 18–38. *Source: Cox* et al. *(1993), Table 2.17, p. 31.*

The overall rates of alcohol consumption are very similar in the two surveys but there is a great deal of change in individuals' behaviour.

There were, however, some areas where there were significant changes in the seven years between HALS1 and HALS2: there was an increase in the use of medication among all age groups and social classes; there was an increase in the prevalence of those overweight. Changes in behaviour to promote health including more exercise and better diet were shown for men aged 45 and above, but not for men below this age.

Concepts of health

In HALS1 respondents were asked two questions about their concepts of health:

(1) Think of someone you know who is very healthy... What makes you call them healthy?

(2)   At times people are healthier than at other times. What is it like when you are healthy?

The replies were written down verbatim and later coded. The main categories were: never ill, physical fitness, functionally able, psychologically fit (Figure 4.7).

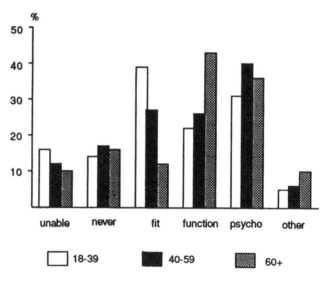

Figure 4.7   Concepts of health for men by age. *Source: Blaxter, 1990 Table 3.2, p. 18.*

Younger men tend to speak of health in terms of physical strength and fitness whereas younger women favour ideas of energy, vitality and ability to cope. Older people, particularly men, think of health in terms of function, or the ability to do things. At all ages men give less expansive answers than women who appeared to find the question more interesting. Few men included social relationships in their definition of health.

Class and small area

An interesting finding from the examination of small area 'families' is that class is related in different ways in different types of area. There was little difference in smoking behaviour in men between non-manual and manual classes in rural or resort and retirement areas, whereas there were significant differences in high status, industrial, local authority housing, and cities and inner and central London (Figure 4.8).

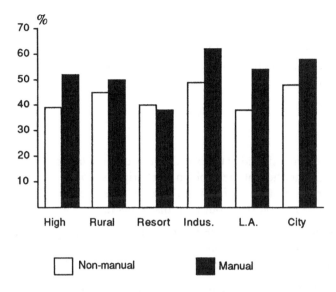

Figure 4.8 Smoking by class in small areas. *Source: Blaxter, 1990, Table 6.3, p. 117.*

Some conclusions

Few people's lifestyles are totally healthy (15%) or unhealthy (5%) in all four areas of life examined, smoking, alcohol consumption, diet and exercise: most are mixed.

It is in the middle years of life, particularly for men, that the relationship between social circumstances and health are strongest. The differences between younger adults are not so great. Among older men and women health is more equal for the survivors.

Alcohol

In 1990, the cost to UK industry of deaths from alcoholism was £1.3 billion (Long, 1991). Goddard (1991) explores the debate that the effects of drinking can be both positive and negative, and argues that the high mortality or prevalence of illness amongst abstainers could be due to previous drinking patterns.

Many organisations who in the past condoned drinking of alcohol as part of a person's occupation, now have very definite policies on workplace drinking. Most breweries are now 'dry' workplaces, where alcohol for consumption by employees is banned. Other workplaces may have alcohol policies in relation to drinking on the organisation's premises, but there is the fact that employees could drink alcohol during their lunch break and return to work for the afternoon. Goddard (1991) found a direct association between social class and drinking during working hours. The association was not the common one that people normally make: those in social class I were much more likely to take a drink during working hours than those in social class V.

Sleep

Sleep is rarely mentioned in the health literature in relation to health. There is no specific mention of the topic in Cartwright's review of health surveys (1983), nor in Smith and Jacobson's book, *The Nation's Health* (1988). Blaxter does mention sleep but then discounts it:

> the association of current health and current sleeping habits is so strong that the use of sleeping habits as another 'voluntary behaviour' (in a survey of one moment of time) does not appear to be justified. (Blaxter, 1990, p. 127)

The assumption is that there is already a strongly associated link.

A look through the indexes of books on health would not reveal sleep as a listed category (Currier and Stacey, 1986; Townsend and Davidson, 1982; McDowell and Newell, 1987). In McDowell and Newell's *Measuring Health*, of the measures and scales included, the following include references to sleep:

(1) Functional disability and handicap: no mention.
(2) Psychological well-being:
    (a) health opinion survey;
    (b) the 22 item screening score of psychiatric symptoms;
    (c) the general well-being schedule;
    (d) the general health questionnaire.
(3) Social health: no mention.
(4) Quality of life and life satisfaction: the Philadelphia geriatric centre morale scale.
(5) Pain measurement:
    (a) the Oswestry low back pain disability questionnaire;
    (b) the McGill Pain Questionnaire;
    (c) the pain and distress scale;
    (d) the illness behaviour questionnaire.
(6) General health measurement: the Nottingham Health Profile.

All these scales and measures contain questions or statements which elicit information about an individual's sleep.

Hyyppa (1991) suggests that when considering strategies of sleep, promotion and counselling need to be substantiated with scientific data rather than subjective and cultural approaches. There are suggestions that good sleepers seem to demonstrate qualities and attributes consistent with good or positive mental health.

Berrios and Shapiro (1993) feel that:

> About a third of people who go to see their general practitioners and about two thirds of those who see psychiatrists complain that they are dissatisfied with the restorative quality of their sleep... Despite the size of these groups and the advances made by research workers, practical knowledge about the diagnosis and management of sleep related complaints is limited. (p. 843)

Berrios and Shapiro feel that medical schools provide inadequate teaching about sleep disorders, and that many doctors hold the same beliefs about sleep disorders as their patients. These are often unsubstantiated and are thought to be secondary to some other condition or event. They feel that patients often blame recently developed fatigue, depression, irritability, tension, sleepiness, lack of concentration, drowsiness or muscular aches on the quality of their sleep. Sleep therefore is seen as important to individuals, but probably only as an indication of something else.

In a study by Jacquinet-Salord, *et al.* (1993), on sleeping tablet consumption, self reported quality of sleep, and working conditions, the following conclusions were drawn:

> A high prevalence of self reported sleep problems and related drug consumption was observed. Physical working conditions were not related to the quality of sleep in contrast to perceived job conditions. The results suggest that sleep quality might be a useful health indicator for the occupational physician. (p. 64)

This study was undertaken in 2769 small to medium sized firms in the Paris area. The study found no association between working conditions and sleep disturbances and drug consumption. The study was a large one, with a random sample of 7629 employees, 61% men and 39% women. People assessed their own quality of sleep; 16% of men and 26% of women said that they had sleep disturbances. One of the main reasons that people in this study took sleeping tablets was because of 'bad atmosphere at work'.

Illness

As a result of their research, Morse and Johnson (1991, p. 317) have developed an illness-constellation model: Figure 4.9. In this model, illness is seen 'as an experience that affects the sick person and his or her significant others'.

Morse and Johnson (1991) feel strongly that theories of illness must be developed from 'the patient's perspective rather than from the perspective of the health care provider, social worker, or significant others' (p. 3). It is

self	others
stage 1 - the stage of uncertainty	
suspecting	suspecting
reading the body	monitoring
being overwhelmed	being overwhelmed
stage 2 - the stage of disruption	
relinquishing control	accepting responsibility
distancing oneself	being vigilant
stage 3 - striving to regain self	
making sense	committing to the struggle
preserving self	buffering
renegotiating roles	renegotiating roles
setting goals	monitoring activities
seeking reassurance	supporting
stage 4 - regaining wellness	
taking charge	relinquishing control
attaining mastery	making it through
seeking closure	seeking closure

Figure 4.9   Illness-constellation model. *Source: Morse and Johnson, 1991, p. 321.*

important to understand how that person feels and thinks in relation to what is happening to him, how he puts that into context of his life, his experiences and his future aspirations.

The usefulness of the illness constellation model is that it views the individual and his experience of illness together with his significant other. It is very rare for a person not to have a significant other at all, and the work that has to be done during illness is a partnership between the person who is ill, their significant other and the health care provider. This model allows for those relationships to be explored and new thinking to emerge.

Summary

In this chapter we have concentrated on developing frameworks for understanding the relationship of masculinities to men's health and illness behaviour. The most significant social and political perspective is provided by Wilkinson's (1996) explanation of health and social capital to which we have applied analysis in terms of gender. The research on the health of black and Asian minority ethnic groups has shown the sensitivity of poverty and standards of living within the broad occupational classes. Further evidence of diversity has been shown by the mental health of Irish people who are often assumed to be part of the undifferentiated white majority.

Research on 'lifestyle' has concentrated on diet, smoking, alcohol, and exercise. We have tried to show that underlying lifestyle are attitudes to risk which are also important with respect to sexual behaviour, and to violence and joy-riding.

Important determinants of gender socialisation which we have not covered are the transmission of attitudes through popular culture (McKibbin, 1998) and through formal education.

Further reading

Blaxter, M. (1990) *Health and Lifestyles*. Tavistock, London.
  This book provides a readable account of the largest national survey of lifestyle. It provides explanations of behaviour in terms of gender and class, but not ethnicity.
Busfield, J. (1996) *Men, Women and Madness. Understanding gender and mental disorder*. Macmillan, Basingstoke.
  Despite the title there is far more emphasis on women and madness. Nevertheless it does help to move the debate onto a social explanation of mental distress rather than a medical explanation of mental illness.
Nazroo, J. Y. (1997a) *The Health of Britain's Ethnic Minorities*. Policy Studies Institute, London.
Nazroo, J. Y. (1997b) *The Mental Health of Ethnic Minorities*. Policy Studies Institute, London.
  These are two reports from the Policy Studies Institute's Fourth National Survey which included health for the first time. It is essential reading on the topic of ethnicity and health.
Wellings, K., Field, J., Johnson, A. and Wadsworth, J. with Bradshaw, S. (1994) *Sexual Health Behaviour in Britain: the National Survey of Sexual Attitudes and Lifestyles*. Penguin, Harmondsworth.
  This is the popular report of the national survey of sexual attitudes and behaviour. It helps to explode many myths, and indicates some aspects where there are significant generational changes.
Wilkinson, R. (1996) *Unhealthy Societies*. Routledge, London.
  Wilkinson provides the first major progress of the debate on inequalities in health since the Black report. The emphasis on health and social capital is very important but he pays little attention to the influence of gender.

Chapter 5
The Health of Men at Work

In this chapter we:

- explore the concept of work in men's lives;
- consider the effects of work on health for men;
- consider the effects of health on work for men;
- describe some of the systems of protection;
- set out the issues to be considered in relation to occupational health and public health.

Introduction

This chapter is about the effects of health on work and of work on health. Wherever possible the issues have been genderised, but this is neither always possible nor desirable. Because of men's traditional role in the workplace much of the occupational disease information relates only to men in that they had the exposure, contracted the disease and became unwell, incapacitated and died. There are graphic historical examples to illustrate this: mule spinner's cancer; scrotal cancer in male workers in the textile industry caused by constant and repeated exposure to mineral oils; coal miners' pneumoconiosis and solidification of men's lungs through the inhalation of coal dust by men working underground in coal mines.

In some industries where both men and women were exposed, then both contracted occupational diseases: asbestosis and mesothelioma of the lung in the asbestos industry; bysinosis in the cotton industry. Men and women are equally vulnerable to occupational dermatitis and occupational asthma. It is a question of opportunity, exposure and individual susceptibility.

The place of work in men's lives

Concepts of work

For centuries it has been acknowledged that work can have an effect on health, either positive or negative. The positive effects include social position, active occupation, and freedom from poverty and utilisation of knowledge and skills. An ability to contribute to a community is often seen by some people as a justifiable basis for working. Working is and has been an acceptable aspect of our culture. In the future it may be necessary to rethink this strongly held belief. There may not be sufficient traditional work for everyone, and as long as society holds the view that people should contribute to society by formal work, there will be conflict.

Watson (1987) sees work as: 'Carrying out of tasks which enable people to make a living within the environment in which they find themselves' (p. 83).

When considering the history of work in society it is important to remember time and context. Slaves may not have gained much by their ability to work beyond staying alive. Many views were expressed about the value of work: a Protestant work ethic was seen as a 'good thing' until work was either not available or people were not able to perform their work, then of course they were at fault. There are a range of views held about work today, some positive, some negative, and many politically motivated.

The early social scientists developed theories on the place and effect of work in society. These views were based on individual values and beliefs and would explore aspects of that individual's culture, experience and exposure (Sennett, 1998). The same could be said of each individual in society; their views of work and leisure are personal, idiosyncratic and value laden, and may or may not have changed since the mid 1980s. Questions are being raised about the whole notion of existing work patterns and the concept of work (Handy, 1989). This change in thinking is related to the changing employment market and the emergence of technology and its effect on the labour force. Handy raises the notion of wage work, fee work, gift work and study work. This is a difficult transition for many people who have been raised on the Protestant work ethic to make, and requires a different way of thinking. A person may not be paid for some of this work; that is not usually why people do work. It may mean that people will need to be paid more for the smaller proportion of formal, i.e. wage work that they do.

The social evils associated with some occupations have been graphically described in novels through the ages. The Victorian novelists, particularly, used their books to describe the ills of their times, but before then in the 1700s Bernadino Ramazzini described the ills of working in certain trades and occupations.

> ... we must admit that the workers in certain arts and crafts sometimes derive from them grave injuries, so that where they hoped for a subsistence that would prolong their lives and feed their families, they are too often repaid with the most dangerous diseases, and finally, uttering curses on the profession to which they have devoted themselves, they desert their post among the living. (Ramazzini, 1713, p. 7)

There has probably never been such a change in working lives as there is now. During the lifetime of the authors of this book, the changes in society have been phenomenal. Work, even so little as 20 years ago, carried with it an expectation of routine, a predictability:

> ... though he was only forty when I first met him, Enrico knew precisely when he would retire and how much money he would have. (Sennett, 1998, p. 16)

Sennett says that for him one of the most tangible signs of change is the motto 'No long term'. This leads to expectations of a work force that will be responsive and flexible, not only about the work they do, but where they will do that work. There is a loss of 'self' in relation to work.

The range of work done by men

Since the industrial revolution until quite recently work, and particularly work that men do, has been outside the home. There has been an acute division between men's work and women's work. In the UK working age is 16–65 years for men and 16–60 years for women, and in 1993 the number of people at work stood at 34.6 million. It is however, more usual to calculate the labour force, that is the number of people over 16 'in the economy in work or available for work' (Drever, 1995, p. 16). In 1993, the labour force stood at 27.1 million. There has been a considerable increase of women in the labour force (of an increase of 3.2 million since 1973, 2.8 million is accounted for by women). Male activity rates for men between 1973 and 1993 fell from 90% to 85%, female activity rates rose from 59% to 71%.

These changes are thought to be due to higher proportion of women entering the labour market, increased availability of part time work, and changing social attitudes. For men the issues are different, there appears to be a higher proportion of men taking early retirement (do they go or are they pushed?), changes away from traditional male-dominated industries (coal, metal, engineering). It is not just older males who are no longer in employment, 'prime age males' i.e. 25–44 years old have also had a fall in activity rates.

The demand for labour has also changed, employment in the manufacturing sector has fallen since 1973 from 32% to 19% in 1993 and in the services sector it has risen from 55% in 1973 to 71% in 1993. The service sector is not a traditional male employment area. So men's jobs are changing or going out of existence; what does this mean for men and work in the future? We have a culture which values 'strong' men, both emotionally and physically; where will we go with this in the future? There are now examples of men moving into traditional female areas of work. In Sheffield, half of the city's childcare centre carers are men (McClarence,

1998). This leads to an interesting debate about role, gender and place in society, particularly as some of these men used to be steelworkers.

Effects of work on health

Work can affect people in many ways. Harm can be done to people by the work that they do.

> One particularly striking way in which an individual's social background can [cause] disease and death is through the effects of working in a particular occupation. (Tuckett, 1976, p. 110)

Other people are affected by a combination of factors, their work exposure to substances which can cause ill health or disease, such as lead, asbestos, noise and alcohol, together with work practices such as shift working and job stress. Over and above this is the possibility of personal and social demands, which could become stressors. In 1995 it was estimated that 2 million people in the UK suffered from an illness which *they* believed was caused by their work, and an estimated 19.5 million working days were lost because of work-related illness (HSC, 1998).

Sickness absence is a multifactorial issue, not necessarily related to sickness, but using sickness as a legitimising reason for not being at work. Women have a higher rate of sickness absence than men, with more short-term absences than men. Women however, report fewer health problems which 'limit their work' (Clarke *et al.*, 1995). When the data for sickness absence are further analysed, the majority of absences are for 1–3 days, self certification of absence from work may affect reporting in this category,

> As well as responsibilities outside the working environment... Other factors such as job dissatisfaction, stress or lack of general well being may increase the relative incidence of short-term absence. (Clarke *et al.*, 1995, p. 228)

Work limiting health conditions in the working population generally are musculoskeletal problems, respiratory disease and cardiovascular disorders. It is strongly felt that social and economic factors are at play in this area with lower socio-economic status having a greater percentage of work limiting health conditions.

In 1998 the Health and Safety Commission/Executive (HSC/E) launched a consultative document aimed at identifying a strategy for occupational health in the UK for the next ten years (HSE, 1998a). HSC/E see this document as an opportunity to identify and promote partnerships. They see themselves as ensuring that workplace activities are controlled. They see other partners being involved in 'treatment, prevention, rehabilitation and promotion' (p. 3). This document identifies a very changed working population within the currency of the study: fewer people employed in manufacturing and more in the service sector; more people being employed part time or being self-employed; more small firms; more women in employment; an older workforce; teleworking; and people regularly changing their jobs rather than having a job for life. This changing population will mean that there is need to think about how the health of people at work can be sensibly managed. Old methods and systems will not meet the need, new thinking is required, but not necessarily self-regulation.

There has been considerable work completed by epidemiologists on the effects of work on health and health on work (WHO, 1986a). This work has in the main been substance specific, i.e. focusing on lead workers or asbestos workers, rather than a general overview of workers' health (Townsend and Davidson, 1982). This is probably because of the volume, i.e. number of people affected. With improved technology it has also become easier to manage and control the working environment, and so targeting a particular substance provides a focus. The assumption remains that a person who works is 'healthy' by virtue of being at work, and the health of the employed population has not been considered an issue of public health in the recent past (DHSS, 1988).

Occupational disease and accidents

We know how many people are killed in the workplace each year, the number for 1997/98 is 268 (HSC, 1998). This includes both employed and self-employed individuals. The major cause of fatal accidents was 'falling from heights' (Drever, 1995). Minor injuries often go unrecorded, and without appropriate treatment and care could progress to more serious conditions. We do not really know how many people die as a result of occupational disease, diseases that are attributable to occupation only, although a figure of 750 per year is given by the Central Statistical Office (CSO, 1987). Figures on morbidity and mortality are published by many organisations, the Health and Safety Executive (HSE), Health and Safety Commission (HSC), Office of Population Censuses and Surveys (OPCS), and Central Statistics Office (CSO); but often the basis of the decision making for mortality relies on a death certificate, and these are known to be unreliable in providing morbidity data (Harrington & Seaton, 1988). The death certificates will give causes of death, but may not record all the conditions from which the person suffered. There is a view that many more people may be suffering from diseases attributable to working conditions, which are not prescribed (Royal Commission on Civil Liberties, 1987). The requirements for prescribing a disease are very rigorous and quite specific (DHSS, 1979), and the true incidence of occupational disease in the UK is probably underrated by a factor of two or three (Harrington and Seaton,

1988). So although figures are published they may only be the tip of the iceberg. For example, in 1997/98 there were 1,300 deaths from meso-thelioma, an occupational disease caused by working with asbestos.

In 1990, the OPCS carried out a survey of households for the Department of Employment, the Labour Force Survey (LFS), and included a question on the relationship between work and health. The response must be viewed as a self-reported work-related illness without verification. The highest reported disease groups were: musculoskeletal conditions, with the highest number of problems being associated with back disorders, then came stress and/or depression, then unspecified 'other' diseases, long-term effects of trauma and poisoning and then more or less equally deafness and ear conditions and the lower respiratory diseases (Osman *et al.*, 1995). When the responses are grouped for age and sex, the highest prevalence rates were in the age group 45 years to retirement with 10% for males and 5.8% for females. Male rates were higher in all age groups (Osman *et al.*, 1995).

We do not know the true figures of occupational disease. One of the major problems with morbidity and mortality in occupational disease is the long latent development period, which now can cover a variety of employers. People no longer have a job for life; during a person's occupational lifetime they could have more than one job in more than one organisation, in different parts of the country or even overseas. At one time this would have been only a small group of people who were probably very specialised in what work they did. This is not the case today. Hashemi (1989) attempted to put costs to the problem; he feels that a series of disasters has sensitised us to industrial accidents, but that far more people are killed by occupational disease than industrial accidents. There are figures available for 1996/97 which indicate that there were 116 fatal or major accidents for every 100,000 employees. The latest calculation available (1998) shows that the social costs of work accidents and work related ill health were estimated at between £11 and £16 *billion*. Of this sum, it is calculated that £4–5 billion can be attributed to work related ill health (HSC, 1998). Consider not only the financial and economic costs, but also the personal, social and community costs of this. These costs will not be a once and for all cost, for some people they will continue for the rest of their lives. Managing occupational ill health is the major focus of the HSE occupational health strategy discussion document (HSE, 1998a).

Health hazards associated with work

Hazards at work are classified in the following categories (WHO, 1975):

- chemical;
- physical;

- mechanical;
- biological;
- psychosocial.

This list is used when assessing a workplace for potential hazards.

Substances get into the body by means of inhalation, skin absorption and/ or ingestion. The inhalation of substances is the most common route of entry. The nose usually filters large particles, but small (below 5 microns) particles can enter the alveoli of the lungs from where they can cause local damage or be absorbed into the bloodstream. The skin provides some protection from the absorption of substances, and relatively few substances are directly absorbed, however organic solvents and phenols are. Substances may be absorbed through the skin if it is damaged by injury or disease and not protected. Ingestion of substances is often due to poor personal hygiene, i.e. not washing hands before eating sandwiches, or by nail biting or smoking. There can be instances when inhaled particles are coughed up and are then swallowed. In all instances, there will be individual susceptibility: not all people will respond in the same way to exposure to substances. Susceptibility can depend on age, race, sex, and state of health and level of exposure. Traditionally men have been employed in the more 'dangerous' occupations, legislation to some extent protecting or barring women from exposure.

Chemicals in the workplace can provoke a fairly standard response in individuals. They can cause irritation of the respiratory system, the skin and eyes. There can also be sensitisation of both the respiratory system and the skin.

Long-term effects

There is growing concern that long-term exposure to chemicals can result in cancer. The area of study is fraught with difficulty (Doll, 1985). There are certain groups of workers who have traditionally identified the relationship between exposure and cancer development, i.e. chimney sweeps and mule spinners with scrotal cancer, asbestos workers with lung cancer, outdoor workers with skin cancer. The problem now to be addressed is the multifactorial issues of multiple exposure and occupation.

> At best they (industrialists, trade unionists, officials of regulatory agencies) are bemused by the number of contradictory reports; at worst they ignore signs of important new hazards or undermine harmless industries on which employment and the economic health of society depends (Doll, 1985, p. 23).

This uncertainty arises out of the complex nature of the problem and the difficulties in studying the issues. The multifactorial issues of exposure to substances have been demonstrated in synergistic relationship between just two factors, i.e. smoking and exposure to asbestos. This exposure to two carcinogens increases the risk of cancer considerably (TUC, 1988).

Some substances have an immediate effect causing conditions such as occupational asthma (Dobson, 1989). Others have a medium-term effect, which can of course be variable; this could be the development of skin changes, dermatitis, acne or skin cancer (Waldron, 1977). Long-term effects have been described in men and women whose reproductive health has been affected following exposure to chemicals. Some substances can be teratogenic, having an effect on the foetus. It is thought that the following are teratogenic: cadmium, lead, mercury, organic solvents, some halogenated hydrocarbons, carbon monoxide, anaesthetic gases, oestrogenic compounds, ionising radiation, and carbon disulphide (Anonymous, 1979). Some of these substances are also mutagenic, that is capable of altering the genetic material of a cell, and this alteration is transmitted to subsequent generations of cells. Mutagens include chloroprene, perchloroethylene and vinyl chloride, which are halogenated hydrocarbons; anaesthetic gases; some pesticides; ionising radiation and ethylene oxide.

Reproductive health

The whole issue of reproductive health is an emotive one, women being seen by some to be singled out by having their career choices restricted by legislation. In America, women working for a leading car battery maker had to produce a certificate of infertility from a medical practitioner if they wished to continue working in a 'good' job producing batteries. The argument was that the health of the unborn child could be affected by exposing the mother to lead. This argument did not allow for the prospective 'mother' to be involved in the debate, and the arbitrary decision made by the organisation is now being tested in the courts (Ellicott, 1990). The argument laid before the courts was that the company's action discriminated against some employees on the grounds of sex. The policy did not apply to fertile men, although lead can equally affect males (Scrivenor, 1991).

Stijkel and van Dijk (1995) explore the concept of equality in this emotive area of reproductive health and risk. They argue that where there is a known reproductive risk, the emphasis is on the woman. This is not, of course, always the case. They continue, stating that there are two types of risk: 'the direct risks to the workers, and the indirect risks through the workers to their progeny' (p. 298). Stijkel and van Dijk would like greater consideration to be given to equal rights and equal opportunities within this area of risk, and for all individuals exposed to known and potential hazards at work to have equal consideration.

Barker (1991) gives a strong case that the preconception health of parents is an indicator of health and ill health. This is particularly significant for reducing inequalities in health. There is the need for:

> a new national strategy for reducing inequalities in health in Britain . . . The new one will need to address differences in the growth of babies and in the nutrition and health of their mothers [fathers are not mentioned] . . . the seeds of inequalities in health in the next century are being sown today. (Barker, 1991, p. 67)

There has been limited research on the effects of paternal contribution to birth defects, mostly in the USA as a result of concerns about Vietnam veterans exposed to Agent Orange.

> While certain suggestive evidence is reviewed here, conclusive data are yet to be found. Yet, we must remember that it was not long ago that the placenta was assumed to be an impenetrable barrier between mother and foetus. (Cohen, 1986, p. 62)

There is growing epidemiological evidence of associations between male exposures to exogenous agents and abnormal reproductive outcomes (fetal loss, birth defects, childhood cancer, etc.) (Wyrobek, 1993). There is more recent interest in Britain as a result of anxiety about effects of chemical weapons in the Gulf war.

Work environment

Men have traditionally done work which was harder, and more physically demanding, although some women would argue this point particularly in occupations such as nursing. This group would cover activities in the workplace, which could have an effect on an individual in a physical sense; this could include accidents such as tripping over objects, objects falling onto people, slipping on a wet or greasy floor. Other areas of concern would be repetitive strain injury, muscular injury, problems associated with working posture, working in confined spaces or carrying out work which requires employees to wear protective clothing and equipment.

Olsen and Kristensen (1991), in a study in Denmark which addressed the impact of work environment on cardiovascular diseases, describe how physical exercise has to be both vigorous and dynamic if it is to be contributing to the reduction in cardiovascular disease. They feel that only postmen and ballet dancers would be found to have sufficient dynamic muscle work. These authors feel that only 10% of the Danish work force have enough dynamic and aerobic muscle work during working hours. The occupational patterns in the UK are not dissimilar to those in Denmark, so the same problems probably exist.

Mechanisation in industry has brought with it the problem of noise in the workplace, the resulting deafness being referred to as 'occupational induced hearing loss' for which benefit is paid. Repetitive strain injuries are described as the disease of the 1980s and after. We ask people to wear protective clothing and equipment to do their work: eye protection (Banerjee, 1990), hearing defenders, respirators, breathing equipment, gloves, helmets, protective suits and shoes. Sometimes the 'protective clothing' which is provided becomes a contributory factor in accidental injury. Mechanical hazards would be linked to occupations where there is a potential for damage by mechanical means. Equipment in the workplace can be a cause of hazard if it is not guarded adequately or guards are removed. Equipment is sometimes given more care and attention in a workplace than the people who work with the equipment.

Any form of work which results in people coming into contact with biological substances has the potential for hazard. This group of workers would range from chefs in up-market restaurants through market traders selling fruit and vegetables through farmers to microbiologists in hospital laboratories. The range of work is very extensive. In addition to the more straightforward infection hazards, people can develop allergies and sensitivities to biological substances. Equally, a bull could gore a farmer.

There are many hazards which could affect a worker from a psychological and/or social point of view, but which stem from the workplace rather than what the person brings to work with him. Examples would include working unsociable hours, abuse at work, feelings of stress, lack of control in work processes, shift working, or boredom.

There are physical stresses in the workplace which can affect a person psychosocially, e.g. poor visibility, noise, vibration, heat, cold, humidity, wind, motion, perceived dangers, overwork or underload, nightshifts and combinations of these (Poulton, 1978). Blaxter (1990) identifies psychosocial health as one of the four dimensions of health, the other three being unfitness or fitness, disease and impairment or their absence, and experienced illness or freedom from illness. It is important for people at work to be considered as a whole person and for there to be an acknowledgement that their psychosocial health can be affected by the work that they do, equally that factors affecting their psychosocial health away from work can have an effect on the performance at work, i.e. divorce, separation, bereavement, moving house, changing job.

This area of psychosocial hazards is an area of growing concern, and can often be a direct reflection of the nature and culture of an organisation (Hearn, 1993). There are certain occupations which are considered to be 'masculine or male only' jobs. The men in these jobs are also expected to deal with not only hard physical work but also sometimes very emotional work. An example of this could be the emergency services. In the past it was felt that men in these services could 'handle anything', but the emotional trauma of some experiences has left men severely damaged. Almost daily we see examples of disasters and misadventures on the television, and firemen, policemen and ambulancemen (and now women) dealing with these events. A culture which does not acknowledge personal sensitivity to repeated exposure to trauma is in itself flawed and unhealthy (Duckworth, 1991; McCloy, 1992). Fortunately, there is now a change in culture and an understanding that all of us have limits to what can be tolerated.

Management styles in organisations are now being observed, analysed and reported on. This study of organisations has now begun to incorporate issues of gender, and particularly masculinity (Kanter, 1993). Collinson and Hearn (1996) explore in some considerable detail 'men as managers and managers as men'. If the tone or culture of an organisation is masculine and the work itself is masculine, them some employees will have a very difficult time at work. It would appear that some men in management are as 'unkind' [probably a female word] to men in their 'control' as they are to women.

There is increased concern about the effects of aggression, violence and bullying in the workplace. A recent case of a deputy head teacher (male) bullied at work by his head teacher (female) resulted in an out-of-court settlement of £100,000. This is thought to be the first successful stress case by a teacher (Clarke, 1998).

Suicide by certain groups of people has been linked to both employment and unemployment. In relation to employment:

> certain occupations have a higher risk of suicide, and over the period 1979–1990 among men, vets, pharmacists, dentists, farmers and doctors were most at risk. (ONS, 1998, p. 136)

All these occupational groups would, through their employment, have access to the means of committing suicide. In addition, all of them could be called 'small business' men who have to manage a career and run a small business, and probably have to borrow money for investment in the business.

The effects of health on work

It is difficult to identify all existing ill health conditions that people bring with them to the workplace; these can be many and varied. Young people starting work could have conditions which, even if they are not a health issue now, have the potential for being a future problem. For example, a young person with diabetes or a skin condition or an existing lung dysfunction could be put into a job which was not compatible with that condition; it could be aggravated or exacerbated. A person with diabetes could have difficulty working shifts; they need to be able to manage their diet properly, so an erratic type of working may be a difficulty. Some skin conditions can be aggravated by immersion in liquids or irritated by substances such as solvents. A job with lots of physical activity could be a difficulty for people with an impaired lung function; they may not have the capacity. Equally, people who suffer from asthma could be distressed if exposed to sensitisers in the workplace. Older people, possibly through occupational exposure or general wear and tear, could be feeling the effects of existing ill health conditions; lung conditions, musculoskeletal problems.

Most of the statistical information on health is collected via morbidity and mortality information: medical opinion described through doctors' notes/certificates and death certificates. The implications are that we build up a store of knowledge on negatives of health. We use proxy measures to describe health. Also we have a system which interprets what an individual is experiencing into a medical model of disease. This sort of information is not always helpful, particularly if connections between health and work need to be made. There can be difficulties in identifying the range of occupations a person may have done.

Dermatitis is responsible for 132 000 days absence from work in the UK, affecting 84 000 workers (HSE, 1998b) and yet, the views of Engel and Rycroft (1988) who argued that there was:

> less known about the relationship between skin conditions (dermatoses) and employment than some dermatologists and occupational physicians care to admit (p. 114)

would probably still hold true.

A study in Sweden (Rystedt, 1985) found that the development of dermatitis was not a normal progression, even amongst people who had moderate or severe atopic childhood eczema, when exposed to high risk jobs in industry. It does seem, therefore, unfair to label and exclude someone from an activity on the basis of our current notions of health; rather we should be treating each person as an individual. This individual will need to be assessed and individual norms established. These will need to be monitored and evaluated. An important element in this process will be documentation and recording of available information. More recent work by HSE has identified specific occupational groups who need consideration particularly in relation to skin care (HSE, 1996 and 1998b).

A longitudinal study of the causes of death of 17 530 civil servants was conducted over a ten year period by Marmot, Shipley and Rose (1984). The aim of the study was to explore social class differences in mortality in a group of men aged 40–64. The men were classified according to occupational grade, i.e. administrative, professional, executive, clerical and 'other'. The men all had an initial screening examination between 1967 and 1969. This examination included the London School of Hygiene Cardiovascular Questionnaire (this questionnaire is not discussed in the article) and questions on smoking history, respiratory system, medical treatment and leisure-time activities. There was also a physical examination which included electrocardiograms, estimation of blood pressure, plasma cholesterol, post-load blood glucose, skin fold thickness, height and weight ratios. The individuals' NHS records were identified and a copy of death certificates obtained for those men who had died within the UK following this examination.

The results identified that the lower the employment grade, the higher was the mortality for coronary heart disease (CHD). The researchers found a three-fold difference between lowest and highest employment grades in the civil service; this was in the same direction as national differences, but much greater. The men included in the study were all in stable, sedentary jobs in London and not exposed to industrial hazards. It was found that smoking was more common in the lower grades, and this is now firmly linked to CHD (HEA, 1991; Doll and Peto, 1981; Smith and Jacobson, 1988). Marmot et al. (1984) went on to speculate that social class and early life effects, housing, diet, father's occupation, were an important consideration. This view has since been substantiated by the work of Barker (1991) who has explored 'the foetal and infant origins of inequalities in health in Britain'. Barker found a north/south divide, and that this was related to diet and social class.

A second study of 10 314 civil servants (6900 men and 3414 women aged between 35–55 during 1985 to 1988) by Marmot et al. (1991) found similar patterns to the earlier study in relation to social class and morbidity. The researchers found that perceptions of health status and symptoms were worse in people who held lower status jobs. They concluded that there needed to be an encouragement of healthy behaviours across society, and more attention needed to be paid to social environments, job design and the consequences of income inequality. An important feature in this area of research is the concept of control and how much control individuals at work feel they have over both their working life and life in general. Although the working arrangements described in these two previous studies have changed considerably, and therefore some elements of the research may not be applicable now, this central concept of personal control is still an important one.

Illness can be seen by some people as something outside their control; this is described in the literature as 'locus of control' (Niven, 1989). Niven describes the work of Rotter (1954) who developed a series of statements which indicated whether a person had an internal or external locus of control. People with an external locus of control feel that they are not in charge of their fate and that outside forces such as luck or destiny can affect their health and life events. People with an internal locus of control are more likely to feel they have the ability to influence and determine events.

Calnan (1988) used a development of the health locus of control model which focuses on multidimensional health locus of control. The model consisted of three dimensions of belief about the source of control of health: internal, powerful other and chance. High internal scores relate to individual behaviour, while high scores on the other two dimensions relate to lack of personal control. Calnan looked at three aspects of behaviour: cigarette smoking, drinking alcohol and levels of physical exercise. The level of relationship identified was, in Calnan's words, 'never more than modest' (p. 326). One result was more positive:

> The strongest relationship, however, was between smoking and alcohol: smokers were more likely also to drink. People with high levels of exercise were also more likely to be drinkers but were less likely to smoke. (Calnan, 1988, p. 326)

Exercise was the one form of behaviour which was most consistently associated with individuals' beliefs about the locus of control in health. The author feels that beliefs about control over health may be related more directly to certain age groups or social classes, but also that age, gender and education may be confounding the relationships between beliefs and behaviour.

Although Calnan collected information on gender, there was nothing of significance in terms of differentials to report. On all the levels of belief there was no significant difference between males and females. Both male and female respondents had higher scores for 'internal' control as a belief than 'chance' and 'powerful other' (Calnan, 1988, p. 326).

There is a continuing interest in trying to identify aspects of health behaviours and beliefs as a basis for assessing how to target information to affect health behaviours positively (Pietila, 1994 and 1998; Kehoe and Katz, 1998).

Systems of protection

The delivery of occupational health care in the UK is outside the remit of the National Health Service (NHS), although the NHS does provide occupational health services for its staff. The responsibility for the assessment of need and development of policy in relation to the work/health interaction rests with the Health and Safety Commission (HSC) of the Department for Education and Employment. There is no legal obligation on employers to provide for the health of employees at work other than the provision of first aid at work (HSE, 1981), the provision of statutory medical examinations for people exposed to certain substances and procedures (Edwards and McCallum, 1988), and the Control of Substances Hazardous to Health Regulations 1994 and 1996.

Legislative framework

Historically the legal framework surrounding work and health was developed first of all for children, then for women and young people, and men came latterly into the frame through such actions as the Workmen's Compensation Act 1897. This act established the principle, irrespective of negligence, of the employer's responsibility for the payment of compensation (Hunter, 1959).

Health and safety legislation developed on an industry specific basis, dealing with the particular needs of the various industries. This meant that some industries were outside legislative control. Examples of these were the NHS, the education sector and local authorities. During the late 1960s and early 1970s there was considerable concern for the very high accident rate among the working population. There was also a very high rate of mortality and morbidity due to occupational disease. A committee, chaired by Lord Robens, produced a report in 1972 (Department of Employment, 1972), which resulted in the Health and Safety at Work Act 1974 (HSAWA). This act covered all people at work, except domestic workers in private employment. It is an enabling act which has allowed for changes in need to be dealt with much easier through the production of approved Codes of Practice rather than specific regulations and Acts of Parliament. This development can be seen in the programme of developments of such Approved Codes of Practice as those for First Aid (1981), and the Codes developed out of the Control of Substances Hazardous to Health (COSHH) regulations.

The HSAWA is criminal legislation and prosecutions are heard through the magistrates' courts or the crown courts. Offenders can receive fines or be sent to prison.

Recording of occupational accidents and ill health

Prescribed industrial diseases were first described in the Disabled Persons (Employment) Act 1944 which listed diseases for which people would receive financial compensation for loss of physical or mental faculty arising out of work activity:

> (a person) who on account of injury, disease or congenital deformity is substantially handicapped in getting or keeping suitable employment at work. (West, 1962)

The title has now changed to recordable diseases (HSE, 1985) and includes a total of 28 specific conditions in the broad groupings of 'poisoning, skin diseases, lung diseases, infections and a group of miscellaneous diseases which are associated with exposure to particular chemicals or physical agents' (The Reporting of Injuries, Diseases and Dangerous Occurrences Regulations (RIDDOR), 1985) (HSE, 1986). There has still to be a link with work activity and compensation is dependent on medical diagnoses. Depending on medical diagnosis can have limitations, in that the degree of disease present will affect the ability of medical practitioners to make a diagnosis. Although diagnostic skills have improved tremendously, there is perhaps still a time when all the 'signs' are not there to be observed, the person is still feeling unwell or tired or dysfunctional in some way.

Health care in the workplace

Occupational health (OH) is the care of the health of people at work. The WHO produced a definition of occupational health:

(1) To identify and bring under control at the workplace all chemical, physical, mechanical, biological and psychosocial agents that are known to be or suspected of being hazardous;
(2) to ensure that the physical and mental demands imposed on people at work by their respective jobs are properly matched with their individual anatomical, physiological and psychological capabilities, needs and limitations;
(3) to provide effective measures to protect those who are especially vulnerable to adverse working conditions. (WHO, 1975)

In order to comply with the WHO definition of occupational health, there needs to be some understanding of how those needs will be met.

A difficulty in the provision of health care in the workplace, and as such any uniform overview, is the lack of provision of occupational health services (OHS). The UK is one of the few countries in the European Economic Community (EEC) which does not have a policy statement on occupational health. Up to half of the workforce in Great Britain has little or no regular access to occupational health advice (HSE, 1985). In the main, where employers provide OHS in the UK, their provision is voluntary. The range and number of occupational health services is proof that employers see the value of having such a service for their employees. Philanthropic employers who saw the need to provide for the health care of employees developed the early OHS. These services tended to be in larger organisations, this is still the same today with small and medium-sized organisations not having access to OHS.

Occupational health is therefore voluntary, and not a feature of national health provision. This means that all people who work do not have access to an occupational health service. When there is a need to consider their individual work/health relationship they could be disadvantaged by being cared for by health professionals who do not have an appreciation of the effect of work on health for that individual, and could possibly be given inappropriate or unsafe advice. Many providers of health care may not know to ask questions about 'chemical, physical, mechanical, biological or psychosocial agents' (WHO, 1975) to which a person could be exposed in the workplace. They may know little or nothing about the physical or mental demands of a job, and even less about methods of prevention or protection.

Trade union and employee representative involvement

There is also a strong tradition of worker involvement in health and safety issues in the workplace through the activities of trade unions. There is a long history of effective action in reducing the risks associated with the effects of work on health. At the annual Trades Union Congress (TUC) in Blackpool in September 1987, the TUC re-affirmed its intention to play a central role in protecting people from hazards of their work (TUC, 1988). The ultimate responsibility rests with the employer or owner of the organisation, but trade unionists see that they have a part to play not only in working with local employers and industrial groups but also at a governmental level.

The health problems associated with work are still occurring, and although employers and trade unions in many instances have made incredible strides to resolve these problems, they are still with us. People at work are still being damaged, and the underlying philosophy in the UK is one of self-regulation.

Public health and occupational health

Health at work should not be divorced from mainstream health issues, as the two are closely interrelated. The effects of work on health have been documented for centuries. To distance these effects from other health issues produces a false and unrealistic view of a nation's health. It also presents real difficulties when attempting to control or prevent poor health in the workplace. The NHS often has to deal with the end product of health being affected by work. This may be the result of trauma and injury, occupational disease, or mental ill health caused by stress and tension at work. Regulation is not the full answer. Workplaces could be made the safest of places, but there would be no work being carried on. Regulation is important to set the standards, and inspection to ensure the standards are kept, but there also needs to be compliance and co-operation by people who come into the workplace, a sharing of responsibility to care for each other. What is required is a shift in philosophy: work needs to be seen as a potential influence on health. There needs to be a shared sense of responsibility. This will require more comprehensive education of health care professionals to make care of people at work an integrated activity in the community. The work a person does has the potential to reward that individual and make them fulfilled, and also to damage them. To ask the relevant questions, health professionals need to have their awareness raised, their knowledge base improved, their skills refined and their attitudes modified.

There is now a move in the UK to consider seriously occupational health as an element of the public health. The present government's publication 'Our Healthier Nation' (DOH, 1998a) is a consultation paper on public health which identifies three settings for action:

- healthy schools – focus on children;
- healthy workplaces – focus on adults;
- healthy neighbourhoods – focus on older people (p. 6).

In looking at factors affecting health, the paper identifies various areas for consideration. There are fixed factors such genes, sex and ageing. There are social and economic factors, such as poverty, employment and social exclusion. Environmental factors include air quality, housing, water quality and the social environment. Lifestyle is identified as a significant factor and includes diet, physical activity, smoking, alcohol, sexual behaviour and drugs. The final list of factors covers access to services, including education, health services, social services, transport and leisure.

Employment is a key issue:

> Being in work is good for your health. Joblessness has been clearly linked to poor physical and mental health . . . Those in work tend to live longer lives than those without jobs. Unemployed men and women are more likely than people in work to die from cancer, heart disease, accidents and suicide. Losing his job doubles the chances of a middle-aged man dying within the next five years. (DOH, 1998a, p. 17, quoting Drever and Whitehead, 1997)

Social exclusion through unemployment is an equally important issue.

Without doubt there is a strong and positive link between occupational health and public health. One of the biggest challenges in the future will be the ability to make sensible linkages between the people at work and the delivery of primary care. There have been some consideration of these ideas recently (WHO, 1986b; Griffin, 1992; Bamford, 1993 and 1996). Men's health as an element of public health should now extend into occupational health and hence into the variety of workplaces across the UK.

Summary

In this chapter we have shown that there are recent radical changes in the structure of work which are having a major effect upon masculinities because men's identification has been so identified with their work, particularly with heavy manual work. Some of these changes may have a positive effect on men's health such as the involvement of men in childcare which may encourage more emotional honesty and sharing, and other changes may reduce the level of accidents and occupational diseases.

Because so much work used to be clearly divided by gender there had been little explicit attention to the links between gender and health at work. In this chapter we describe the current mechanisms for protection of health at work, and the systems for recording mortality and morbidity. In Chapter 6 we provide some of the limited evidence which is available. Much more research is needed on this subject. Recommendations as to how public and occupational health should be co-ordinated are presented in Chapter 9.

Further reading

Drever, F. (ed.) (1995) *Occupational Health, Decennial Supplement. DS 11.* HMSO, London.
   This is a really comprehensive review of what is happening in the relationship between work and health. It is exceptionally well written and for a publication of this type is very readable.
Health and Safety Commission Annual Reports give year on year accounts of what is happening in relation to health and safety in the workplace.
Sennett, R. (1998) *The Corrosion of Character: the personal consequences of work in the new capitalism.* W.W. Norton & Co., London.
   This book is a must for anyone interested in looking at present day work. It illustrates clearly the changes that have taken place and considers the consequences of changing patterns and behaviours for the individual worker.

Chapter 6
Perceptions of Health Amongst Men at Work

In this chapter we:

- explore some concepts of health and relate them to an employed population;
- consider how this population interfaced with primary care;
- describe how men and women at work articulate their understanding of health;
- illustrate the differences between health professionals' models of care and lay persons' perspectives.

Introduction

This chapter reports on work carried out in 1990–91 in the West Midlands (UK) (Bamford, 1993). The survey was conducted to try to find out what people who are at work, and are therefore presumably well, thought about their health. Although the focus of the research study was not specifically on gender, there is much that can be derived from the findings when we examine similarities and differences between men and women. There has been very little original research on this subject. In Chapter 9 we shall be arguing for both qualitative and quantitative research of this type. This original research needs to be kept up to date, and to be extended to cover a wider sample of organisations. There is also the need to compare working and non-working people.

Table 6.1 shows the age and sex of the respondents to the survey. Table 6.2 shows the organisations and response rates by sex.

Feeling healthy

The people in the survey were asked if they felt they were healthy; overall 92% felt that they were. This figure was similar for men and women, with

Table 6.1 Age and sex of respondents.

age	all number	%	male number	%	female number	%
16–24	43	10	23	8	20	12
25–34	99	22	59	20	40	25
35–44	140	31	92	32	48	29
45–54	117	26	71	25	46	28
55–64	52	12	43	15	9	6
total	451	100	288	100	163	100

Source: Bamford, 1993, p. 157.

slightly more men feeling they were not healthy (22: 8%) than women (7: 2%). This is more positive than Valkonen and Pietiala's (1998) finding in a sample of 250 clients of an occupational health service for the town of Ranua in Finland, where only 62% of the respondents considered themselves healthy. A majority of the respondents in this sample were female, and 93% were in employment or self-employed. It is clear from the lack of literature on the working population and health and wellness, that occupational disease has been the research focus in the past.

There are more general studies around feelings of 'healthiness'. Hanney (1979) found that his sample of Glaswegians considered their health in slightly different categories: 27% felt their health was perfect, 43% good, 22% fair and 5% poor with 2% feeling their health was very poor. The remaining 1% did not have an answer to this question. This could be compared with the employed sample, Table 6.3.

The differences are not that great; Hanney's sample covered a wider age range. It is interesting that both groups had a similar score for the negative element of the response. This was also the same percentage as in the pilot study (Bamford, 1993).

Blaxter (1990), in her study of health and life styles, found that 71% of her respondents defined their health as at least good. The categories they had to choose from were 'good/excellent' and 'fair/poor'.

Reasons for not being healthy

As regards the reasons why people felt they were unhealthy, only a small number emerge, and only 21 of the 33 people gave a reason for feeling unhealthy. The main reason that people felt they were unhealthy was for conditions of the circulation system. This was a very small proportion of the sample, seven people (21%), six men and one woman. A further 12 people (36%) gave no reason for their feelings of not being healthy.

Table 6.2   Organisations in survey and response rates.

	all		male		female	
	response number	response rate %	response number	% by gender	response number	% by gender
emergency service	41	59	37	90	4	10
metal components factory	45	64	39	87	5	11
tyre maker	20	29	20	100	0	0
car components manufacturer	36	51	30	83	5	14
NHS trust	36	51	13	36	23	64
local education authority	34	48	3	9	30	88
L.A. property service	37	53	23	62	14	38
university	32	46	18	56	13	41
electrical components factory	28	40	20	71	8	29
porcelain manufacturer	40	57	22	55	18	45
metal components factory	25	36	20	80	5	20
chemical manufacturer	21	30	11	52	10	48
electrical company	50	71	32	64	18	36
catering company	13	33	1	8	12	92
total	458	47	289	63	165	36

sample = 70 in each organisation (except catering, n = 20)

Source: Bamford, 1993, p. 155.

Table 6.3   Self-rating of healthiness in two surveys.

Bamford		Hanney	
above average	34%	perfect	27%
average	58%	good or fair	65%
below average	7%	poor or very poor	7%

Source: Bamford, 1993, p. 172.

When this group of people are compared with the working class mothers in Pill and Stott's sample (1982), the largest group to emerge are those that used lifestyle as a means of explaining their health (Table 6.4). It can be seen that this understanding related to positive health, i.e. 100 (65%) of the above average health group (n = 155) and only five (38%) of the below average health group (n = 13). When taking the two groups together the percentage for lifestyle is roughly equal at 40% and 42%; a similar pattern emerges for individual susceptibility with 12% and 13%.

Table 6.4   Causes of ill-health by self-assessment of healthiness.

	Pill & Stott	Bamford			
		above average	average	below average	all
germ theory	60%	25%	18%	38%	21%
lifestyle	40%	65%	29%	38%	42%
heredity	34%	1%	0%	0%	0%
stress	20%	7%	3%	23%	5%
environment	15%	2%	2%	15%	3%
individual susceptibility	12%	5%	17%	8%	13%
number	538	160	202	16	378

Source: Bamford, 1993, p. 173.

Germ theory, or the medical model of describing health was used by 96 (21%) of the employed sample against 178 (60%) of Pill and Stott's sample. Pill and Stott argue that their female sample is probably referring to acute short-term illness in this way.

Comparison with others of a similar age

When asked to compare themselves to others of their age, 155 (34%) felt their health was above average, 287 (63%) average, and 13 (3%) felt their health was below average, Figure 6.1.

Of those surveyed, 95 men (33%) and 58 women (35%) felt their health was above average; 173 men (60%) felt their health was average, and roughly half this figure for women, 92 (56%). None of the men who felt they were healthy also felt their health was below average. Of the people who considered themselves healthy, 68 (15%) were worried about their health, and 285 (62%) had worries and anxieties other than their health. In the survey, 82 (18%) of the people who considered themselves healthy had a permanent or long-standing illness, disability or infirmity.

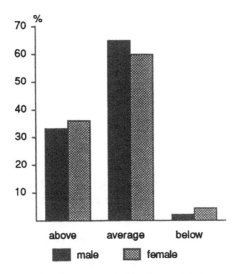

Figure 6.1   Perception of health compared with others of similar age by gender. *Source: Bamford, 1993, p. 174.*

It seems that some people think of average positively and others think of it negatively. Listed below are comments which illustrate this point.

Positive comments:

> I do aerobics and squash most weeks, and have a fairly active job and social life, I don't sit about all day. (female)

> I'm not ill very often, only the usual colds, etc. I lead a very active life at work and at home. (female)

> I can go to work, run a house and go on plenty of walks besides being on my feet all day and getting up at 5 a.m. (female)

> I take tablets for high blood pressure and for Crohn's disease, but I still manage to play rugby and cricket. (male)

Many people who responded in a similar vein, used 'ability to do' as a measure of healthiness or wellness; the absence or control of a condition is also seen as positive.

Negative comments:

> Stress, looking after my father and visiting my mother. (female)

> I tend to have an average life style, without keeping too fit these days. (male)

> Sometimes I feel quite healthy, but a lot of the time I feel tired and sluggish and I'm quite prone to colds. (female)

> Average because don't go out of my way to exercise, etc. Try to eat healthy, but I like my food. (male)

The same concepts are used, but in a way that is negative rather than positive. In both the groups the same ideas and standards are used; the important part is how they are applied.

It is very interesting in this sample to consider the comments that people made to support their numerical score of 2 for health being average when compared to others of a similar age.

Neutral comments:

> I am not as fit physically as some people of my age, but I do not appear to suffer from the disabilities of others in the same group. I therefore consider myself to be of average health overall. (male)

> Some people are obviously fitter, others less so, some with illnesses. (male)

> Some people are better, some worse. (male)

> I visit the doctors occasionally with health problems, the people I know of my age either live at the doctors or never attend, and compared to them I feel that I have an average life. (female)

Neutral comments show that people do make comparisons and judgements and on the basis of these know that they are average.

In this sample, germ theory is the label given to people who use disease and ill-health to explain their health; for example:

> Feel good, suffer no colds, tummy bugs, etc. that others seem to get. (male)

> Because so far I have not suffered from any illness. (male)

This is different from the way that Pill and Stott (1982) use the term, but the underlying principle of illness occurrence is contained in the concept. Some people use the negative of the idea to explain their health, others use the positive:

> I have an active sporting lifestyle, which keeps me fit, but I am prone to minor illnesses, colds, etc. (female)

> I have colds, aches and pains. (female)

> Asthmatic, arthritis in knees, one kidney, lower back pain. (male)

Visiting the doctor

Visits to GPs were given broad bandings of 1–2 months, 3–12 months and 12 months or more, see Figure 6.2. There was a fairly even distribution of

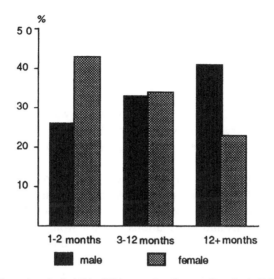

Figure 6.2 Time since last visit to GP by gender. *Source: Bamford, 1993, p. 177.*

attendance across all three groupings when the figures are gender free; however when considered for gender a different picture emerges. In this survey, 70 women (42%) had been to see their GP in the past 1–2 months as opposed to 26% of men. This difference is also reflected at the other end of the scale with 40% of men not having visited their GP in the past year with only 22% of women being in this category.

The distribution of answers to this question is fairly equally distributed between the three groupings of 1–2 months (32%), 3–12 months (33%) and 12+ months (34%). These groupings can be linked to Blaxter's (1985) rating of 1–2 months = high consulters, 3–12 months = average consulters and 12+ months = low consulters. Blaxter's survey was a small-scale survey related to one general practitioner group and included age groups 18+ (a wider age range than this sample of employees). Blaxter found that women were more likely to be high consulters than men, and that men of all ages were likely to be low consulters.

- *Health above average*: in the group who felt their health was above average, 43 people (10%) had visited their doctor during the previous 1–2 months; 46 people (10%) during the previous 3–12 months and 66 (14%) not at all during the previous twelve months.
- *Health average*: in the group who felt their health was average, 41 people (9%) had visited their doctor in the last 1–2 months, 36 (8%) during the last 3–12 months and 20 people (4%) not in the last 12 months.
- *Health below average*: people in this group had a much lower attendance at their doctors. In the 1–2 months prior to filling in the questionnaire, seven (1.5%) had visited their doctor; three people (0.6%) in this group

had visited their doctor in the previous 3–12 months and three people (0.6%) not in the previous twelve months.

Reason for visit

The highest number of visits to GPs by both sexes was for ICD category 8, disorders of respiratory system, with a total of 93 people (20%) seeing their GP with this condition. This was also the highest category for men and women separately.

The next highest category for women was 100. There is no category for prevention in the ICD groupings, so the number 100 was given to cover this category. This would include people visiting their GP for things like health checks, immunisations and vaccinations and for women, birth control. In the survey, 24 women (15%) visited their GP for this preventive activity; there was a slightly lower figure of 13% (37) for men. The second highest reason for men visiting their GP was ICD category 13, disorders of the musculoskeletal systems; 40 men (14%) said this was the reason they had visited their GP.

The next two categories for women were ICD 10, genito-urinary systems, which would include gynaecological conditions with 17 women (10%) visiting for this reason; and ICD 6, nervous systems and sense organs, again with 17 women (10%) visiting. The third highest category for men was category 100, prevention. With the exception of birth control, the reasons for visiting GPs was the same as for women. Some women cited contraception as a medicine they were taking; others did not see this as a form of medicine, but rather a way of not getting pregnant.

Frequency of visits to doctor

In this sample, one third of the group (35%) had not visited their GP in the last twelve months and 110 (24%) had visited their GP only once during the preceding twelve months (Figure 6.3). In 1990 the average number of visits made by individuals of all ages to their GP nationally was five. Males of all ages made four visits per year and females, six visits per year. For males in the age range 16–64 years the national figure would be three, for females in this age range, 5.5 (OPCS, 1992). In this research sample 26% of the men and 9% of women had not seen their GP in the last twelve months; this totalled 35% of the sample (160). Only 1% of each sex had made five visits in the last twelve months. The highest percentage is for one visit in the past twelve months: this is 15% of men and 9% of women. It would appear from the data that there is a lower uptake of GP services amongst this employed population than occurs nationally.

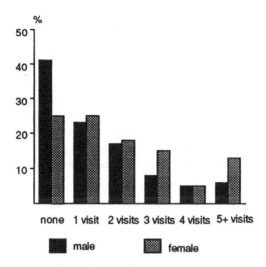

Figure 6.3   Frequency of visits to GP in last 12 months by gender. *Source: Bamford, 1993, p. 181.*

Because of the broader bandings of the OPCS data it is difficult to draw comparisons for all numbers of visits. However, 101 people (63%) aged 16–44 years made no visit to their GP in the last twelve months compared to four visits amongst the national population. For the age range 45–64 years, 58 people (36%) had not made a visit to their GP in the last twelve months (OPCS, 1992).

Disabilities

In this sample, 96 people (21%) identified that they had a permanent or long-standing illness, disability or infirmity, 64 men (22%) and 32 females (19%).

Conditions recorded included the following major categories:

- *Category xiii*: musculoskeletal systems – a total of 28 people recorded a condition in this broad category, 15 men and 13 women. The largest subgroup for both sexes was the group which included 'joints/discs and spines'; conditions fitting into this category included 10 women and 7 men. Other conditions recorded included rheumatism, arthritis, spondylitis and cartilage and muscular problems.
- *Category viii*: respiratory systems – the conditions mentioned by people in this category were all allergy related conditions. Ten people said they had asthma, four hay fever, and three people said they were 'chesty' or allergic to cats, house dust etc.

- *Category vii*: heart and circulation systems – in this category, ten people said they had raised blood pressure or hypertension, five had a cardiac condition or angina, and one person quoted raised blood cholesterol as their long-standing condition.
- *Category ix*: digestive system – here, four people listed an ulcer as their condition, the same number listed conditions of the large bowel, ulcerative colitis, reversed colostomy. Two people had a hernia.
- *Category vi*: nervous system – under this head, three people listed glaucoma, the same number had deafness, two people had epilepsy and one person had visual difficulties; other conditions included nasal rhinitis and sinusitis.

The other conditions listed included 'female conditions' in category x (genito-urinary systems), and three men with diabetes in category iii (endocrine and metabolic systems).

The opportunities to employ people with disability are considerable. The Department for Education and Employment is very supportive to employers and employees alike, offering modification to environments, structures and equipment in the workplace.

Permanent or long-standing illness, disability or infirmity

In the question of the relationship between perception of health and disability, the following results were recorded. Of the group of people who felt their health was above average, 26 people (17%) had a disability, handicap or long-standing illness; 18 men (69%) and eight women (31%).

Medication

The medicine categories being taken at work were recorded and analysed. The highest frequency is in category 2, medicines for cardiovascular disorders, with 26 people (6%) taking this medication. The responses indicated that 104 people (23% of the sample) were taking medication and 98 (21%) of these were taking medication on prescription from their GP. Local pharmacists and workplace surgeries are not major contributors to providing medication.

The non-prescription medicines taken included items such as 'aspirin' taken to prevent coronary heart disease, and cough mixtures and other such substances.

Medication by gender and by perception of health

In the above average health group 21 people (20%) were taking medicine, 77 people (74%) in the average health group and 6 (6%) in the below average group were taking medicine.

When this sample group are looked at for their perception of their health, the largest group of medicine takers are men and women taking medicine for cardiovascular conditions; these people feel their health is average when compared to people of a similar age. The next highest category is men taking medication for pain control.

Other worries

When asked if they worried about things other than their health, 307 people (63%) responded. Of these, 87 (28%) also recorded 'yes' to worries about their health.

The main concerns were contained in a closed question of six categories. People could have responded to more than one answer. The greatest concerns were about employment (24%), worries about money (24%) and family worries (24%). The division between the sexes indicates a raised response in the female group. Females made up just over a third of this sample (36%), and within this questions sample they recorded a 40% response. Collectively employment, money, and family had equal level of worry for both sexes, with well being of least concern for both sexes. The highest level of worry for both sexes was recorded for employment issues, 143 (24%), and this was also the highest level for men. Women were more concerned about family than employment or money, although money came second to family. Men put worries about money second to worries about employment.

The fact that employment and money head this group is not surprising with the West Midlands being in the grip of a recession and many people being made redundant at the time of this survey. Unemployment in the region was approximately 10% at the time of this survey, and people were acutely aware that many large companies were ceasing to trade either through bankruptcy, merger and/or takeover. Mergers and takeovers often result in redundancy and unemployment as 'unprofitable' parts of organisations are closed or rationalised.

It may be that some of these people have already experienced redundancy and unemployment. Of the 146 (49%) who said 'yes' to having worries and anxieties about employment, 87 had done other jobs in their present organisation and 100 had done jobs in other organisations. It is unfortunate that a question on unemployment or redundancy was not included in the questionnaire.

The issue of unemployment and health has been a major focus in the literature during the late 1970s and the 1980s. There seems to be a conscious effort to put distance between the health of the population at large and the employed population. The same philosophy does not apply to the unemployed population, which is much smaller in number and is probably made up of a proportion of people who have been damaged by their work, either disease or injury (Townsend, 1979; Fagin and Little, 1984).

When considering worries other than health, Hanney (1979) identifies four areas of social concern in his study. These were: 'difficulties with children or teenagers, difficulties with other relations, financial difficulties or other problems'. These categories were graded for worry or inconvenience. It would appear from this study of people who are at work that social concerns must include employment, a feature not included by Hanney.

The meaning of 'health'

When people were asked 'What does the word health mean to you?', 94% answered the question, of which 296 responses (69%) included more than one category, i.e. 'physical and mental well being'. 135 responses (31%) included answers such as 'general physical well being', a single factor answer. From the analysis of the respondents' answers it was clear that major themes were emerging, these being: prevention, absence, presence, ability, physical well being, psychological well being and spiritual well being.

The responses that people made to the question: 'What does the word health mean to you?' were compared to a multifaceted concept of health which embraced health, well being, life satisfaction, quality of life and happiness. This proved to be a difficult task, although some statements did fall simply and easily into one of the categories; for example:

- a state of well being (male);
- being healthy (female);
- body working well, feeling good, alert and able to cope (female).

The first statement refers to well being, this is a shorthand statement by which the individual conveys a message about his or her health; with the second statement, by being healthy the person is not unhealthy. The third statement carries three shorthand messages: body working well could mean healthy, feeling good could mean life satisfaction or quality of life, and ability to cope could mean happiness.

One important factor which is not included in this conceptual framework is that of function. This could also be related to strength and/or ability; examples include:

Being responsible for the well-being of my mind and body. Being fully in control by exercising, and eating sensibly and taking note of warning signs. (female)

Well-being, not feeling ill. Being able to do what I want both physically and mentally. I think regular, sensible exercise also contributes to good health. (female)

A complete body/mental/social well-being. Physical fitness, strength, suppleness, stamina linked with emotional, mental well-being and a social confidence. (female)

The notion of 'ability to do' linked to control seems to be a very important concept for people at work. Of the three comments listed above, one is from a senior manager, the other two are from people who would be described as operatives. The statements are no less complex or encompassing.

The meaning of the word 'health' evokes a very personal response by individuals. This response is built up over time and is an outcome of a person's reflection of their life and the lives of other people they have known. It is the sum of their parts. Examples of the allocation of people to categories and 'labels' are given below.

1. Prevention

In bad health some or all of the activities I consider to be normal would be prevented by a physical or mental malfunction. (male)

An increased capability to respond to the flexible demands of life with emphasis placed on prevention. (male)

1.i. Taking care

Looking after yourself. (female)

Your health is something very valuable and it's up to you to take care by eating sensibly, don't smoke, drink alcohol only occasionally. (gender not recorded)

Prevention is better than cure, have smear test, x-ray etc. (female)

1.ii. Avoiding doctors

No pain, no medication, no bloody doctors. (male)

Having an illness and pain free life and not having to visit the doctor too often, either for yourself or family. (male)

1.iii. Environment

Able to lead a full and active life without feeling anything is wrong with oneself and one's family – occupation and environment. (male)

Your health is affected by the lifestyle you presently live and have lived. Health is reliant on a number of things. e.g. exercise, diet, lifestyle, working and home environment. (female)

1.iv. Not to misuse/abuse

Caring for the general well-being of my body by avoiding its misuse or abuse. (sex not recorded)

The word health means to eat and look after your body as well as you possibly can and not to abuse it. (male)

1.v. Avoiding premature death

The maintenance of a body in condition so that life may be enjoyed and the avoidance of premature death. (female)

Long life. (male)

1.vi. Not to be a burden

Being able to do what I want without hesitation and being a liability to other members of my family, friends or colleagues. (male)

The fact that people in this survey used the concept of prevention is an indication that they felt able in some measure to have control of their health and that they could be instrumental in maintaining or enhancing their health by a variety of actions (Currier and Stacey, 1986). People have used positive and negative words to explain their beliefs. If they didn't actively do something then they will be exposing themselves to the possibility of ill-health. One category would fit quite closely to Illich's (1976) perception of the medicalisation of health, 'avoiding doctors'. These persons seem to believe that if they are pain free, take no medicine and have no contact with doctors they will remain healthy. These thoughts seem to be a mix of ideas, perhaps they are generated by what the person has seen happening in colleagues, and in them the result has been ill health. There does seem to be an element of control underpinning these comments. Even where people have used ill health concepts and negative words to describe their beliefs, the emphasis is about them doing something to avoid ill health.

2. Absence

Having no physical or mental disabilities that could change my present way of life. (female)

2.i. Illness

Not suffering from any major illness. (male)

Being well, not ill. (male)

2.ii. Disease/disability

Not having any serious disease/condition and generally being fit within your-self, both physically mentally. (female)

To feel fit, having nothing wrong with you. (male)

2.iii. Pain

Feeling mentally and physically clean, stamina good, relative to age of indi-vidual. Few aches and pains, only those which are self-inflicted; perhaps by sporting activities, nature of your employment. (male)

Being fit, no aches or pains, going where you want and doing what you want. (male)

2.iv. Worries

Being able to lead a reasonably active life-style, dancing, gardening, DIY without having to worry about the effects of the activities on me, able to do my job in an energetic way and get pleasure out of life generally. (male)

2.v. Stress

General well being, good appetite, sleeping well, no stresses, good sex life. (male)

Being fit, average weight, therefore not over weight, strong and healthy, not stressed or anxious. (female)

2.vi. Restrictions

To live life to the full without restriction, to fully support my wife, my company at all times. (male)

2.vii. Medication

Previously quoted in 1.ii: Avoiding doctors.

Absence of conditions or situations which could lead to ill health is a measure of how people are understanding the messages relating to health and ill health. This links in with the medical model; if there is no disease present, i.e. it is absent, then the person is healthy. Worries and stress could be seen as precursors to disease development and therefore ill health. This concept as described by Calnan (1988) would be negative, but the language used by people is both positive and negative. For example, 'to feel fit' (positive); 'having nothing wrong with you' (negative). People generally do not seem to have the same mental divisions as researchers would think they have in viewing their health. Some people are perhaps using language in a different way to others. An example of different use of language is to be found in the next category: Presence.

3. Presence

3.i. Well being

General feeling of well-being, where your everyday life is not adversely affected by ill-health or fitness. (male)

Well-being. (male)

3.ii. Feeling good

Feeling good, being able to carry out tasks to my fullest ability. (male)

Feeling good in myself, a positive outlook on life, fit, able to do all the things I would like to, the feeling that I can go on indefinitely, to eat, sleep, work in a balanced manner. (male)

3.iii. Confidence

Feeling confident and happy and great to be alive. (male)

3.iv. Long life

Longer life. (male)

Feeling good, looking good, being cheerful and trying to live as long as I can. (male)

3.v. Feeling right

It means to me how I feel and how my body feels. (female)

Feeling right with myself, no coughs, colds, aches and pains. (female)

3.vi. Feeling well

Feeling well, clear skin, hair in good condition. (female)

Feeling well and able to cope satisfactorily with modern demands on human life. (male)

3.vii. Feeling healthy

Being healthy. (female)

Feeling good bodily, if one has good health and the reverse if not. (female)

3.viii. Control

Quality of life for yourself, your family around you, well-being, continuity of life on a day to day basis with minimum of unplanned and unwanted instances. (male)

Being of a sound body and mind, being able to live one's life without restrictions and being in complete control. (male)

Presence is more positive than absence. The comments that people made sound more positive, more joyful. In this category, people relate to how they feel: feeling good, feeling confident, feeling right, feeling well, feeling good bodily, feeling right with myself, feeling good in myself. The word is not just related to the individual's physical being, but also to psychological and spiritual being – 'feeling good, looking good, being cheerful'. These people have a personal measure of health which encapsulates this range. There is an element of control in this measure, 'able to do all the things I would like to do' is one way of expressing this, in addition to the use of negative words such as 'unplanned and unwanted', 'without restrictions'. People have also used other negative thoughts to illustrate their thinking, using these as an opposite end of the spectrum, 'no coughs, colds, aches and pains'.

4. Ability

Ability to live and enjoy life. (male)

Ability to carry on, with pleasure, the activities that I wish to do. (male)

4.i. Work

My work. (male)

Looking after myself, wife and kids and being fit to do the job I am employed to do. (male)

4.ii. Play

Not being in pain, fit enough to climb a mountain or hill. (female)

Being able to work and enjoy my leisure time to the full. (male)

4.iii. Function

It means the condition a person may be in and his/her ability to do activities whether it be work or leisure without any restrictions. (male)

The ability to do the things I have to do plus the things I want to do. (male)

4.iv. Care for family

Well being and ability to cope with job, family, home through conscientious monitoring of diet, exercise and relief of stresses. (male)

Looking after myself, eating correctly, regular exercise, making sure my family are OK. (male)

4.v. Responsibility

Being responsible for the well-being of my mind and body, being fully in control by exercising and eating sensibly and taking note of warning signs. (female)

4.vi. Recovery

Feeling of mental and physical well-being, ability to 'shake-off' minor ailments i.e. colds etc. quickly. (female)

'Ability' means to do things, be in control, active, involved, in charge. Perhaps this category more than any other would link to a previous concept held on health, that of strength, not to demonstrate weakness and to feel 'fit' (Williams, 1983). The underlying theme in this section is one of doing, of functioning, and with that an element of control. Even when a negative is used to illustrate, i.e. 'not being in pain', the second part of the individual's thoughts could be classed as heroic, i.e. 'fit enough to climb a mountain or hill'. The mountain comes before the hill, mountains to be climbed now, and when that isn't possible, perhaps a hill.

Also demonstrated in people's ideas is that even where health is about doing, it includes a relationship between physical, psychological and spiritual aspects: being fit to do the job; the ability to do the things I have to do plus the things I want to do; being fully in control; enjoy life; ability to carry on, with pleasure, the activities I wish to do.

5. Physical well-being

Well-being in mind and body. (male)

Physical and mental well-being. (male)

5.i. Exercise

All about the inside of yourself, the way it ticks, due to the food we eat, life we live, exercise we take. (male)

Good health, free of illness, fairly fit, eating and drinking in moderation, keeping fit by walking – lots of fresh air. (female)

5.ii Diet

Looking feeling good, healthy eating, beauty from within one's self, confidence and good skin, hair, eyes and teeth. (female)

Clean life, not to abuse oneself, good steady diet, work and exercise. (female)

5.iii. Relaxation

Being healthy, fit and relaxed (male)

5.iv. Looking good

Feeling good, looking good, being cheerful and trying to live as long as I can. (male)

A good all-round appearance, good all-round fitness. (male)

5.v. Mechanical

All organ and body parts function correctly and completely, consistent with age and normal wear and tear. (male)

5.vi. Energy/vitality/action

Fitness in body and mind, an active life, no illness. (male)

To feel good, fit and active and all bodily functions and systems are working adequately. (male)

5.vii. Lifestyle

Health is feeling of well-being which needs to be looked after in order to lead the life style you want, but not become obsessed with worrying about food etc. (no sex recorded)

To carry on with my work and life-style without recall to my doctor. To carry on leisure time activities without too many repercussions. (no sex recorded)

5.viii. Feeling fit

Feeling and being physically and mentally fit. (male)

Feeling good, looking after yourself, being fit, not out of breath. (male)

Physical wellbeing relates to the mind and body seeming to suggest that people see a balance as being necessary for health. This concept seems to rely on a more mechanical train of thought. There seems to be a relationship in people's minds about inputs and outcomes; what is taken into the body: diet, atmosphere; what is done to the body: exercise, work, bodily function, absence of ill health; together with how the body looks. Perhaps the concept of control is more apparent in this group by means of a more mechanistic approach.

6. Psychological well-being

General well-being and contentment with one's physical and mental state. (male)

The state of one's mind and body. (male)

6.i. Positive attitude

It means everything to me, it is the most important thing in life. (female)

To feel good in body and mind, if you don't have good health, all the money in the world can't buy it for you. Do things in moderation, eat in moderation, too much of anything is no good for us. (female)

6.ii. Ability to cope

Being able to cope with everyday life, without any stress or strain, fit and able to stand up to any physical challenges set for you. (male)

It means being able to be involved in many things and feel good within yourself, I feel if you are healthy then any worries or problems that might occur are not half so bad because you can face them better. (male)

6.iii. Peace of mind

Plenty of energy, peace of mind, a feeling of enjoyment, being able to do things. (male)

Peace of mind and physical condition that permits me to tackle reasonable tasks confidently. (male)

6.iv. Superstition

A good diet, plenty of exercise, a lot of luck, live each day as it comes. (female)

To me the word health means the tightrope that those of us lucky enough to be on, hope we can stay on. Unlike any other kind of tightrope, this depends more on luck than skill. (male)

This section is particularly interesting in that the second highest number of people in the sample (n = 134) made reference to psychological wellbeing, either in the broad category of psychological wellbeing by referring to mind as a component of health, or by means of the subcategories of positive attitude, ability to cope, peace of mind or superstition. Superstition would suggest that the people are assuming they have no control at all of circumstances and situations. This would seem to be even more negative than the 'chance' category described by Calnan (1988).

The other categories move on from the general comments on psychological wellbeing as being the state of one's mind to give examples of how one's mind can affect one's health. The use of stress and strain, worries and problems are negative, but acknowledge that the mind does have an effect on physical well-being.

7. Spiritual well-being

Physical, mental and spiritual well-being. (female)

Health means a good state of mind, body and soul. If you've got a fit mind you will have a fit body and a better attitude to life. (female)

7.i. Enjoying life

Enjoying life without illness, mental or social disorder. (female)

Being able to enjoy life to the full. (female)

7.ii. Fulfilled life/potential

Living. (male)

Being able to enjoy life, feeling physically fit and comfortable; having low stress levels, feeling personally fulfilled in what I do. (male)

7.iii. Quality of life

Quality of life is sufficient for me to carry out my daily tasks unhindered. (female)

Feeling of well-being, which makes the quality of life good. (male)

7.iv. Happiness

Being physically fit in all parts of the body with no pain, stiffness of restrictions, coupled with being mentally happy and active. (male)

Happiness, enjoyment, appreciation, love, thanks, honesty. (male)

7.v. Zest for life

Feeling of well-being and getting on with life. (male)

Feeling confident and happy and great to be alive. (male)

7.vi. Contentment/at ease

Well-being, contented with your work place, and family, but still striving for a bit better. (female)

Living a normal life. (male)

The section on spiritual wellbeing is enormously interesting. People seem to have a feeling for the joy of living which they express in many ways: enjoying life, being fulfilled, having a quality of life, being happy, a zest for living, being content. There is still a use of mixed concepts, positive and negative words, but the essential feeling is one of being uplifted, of strong positive feelings. The comments used to illustrate this section are taken as all comments are from a range of organisations, from all occupational groups and from a cross section of organisational positions.

8. Social well-being

Enjoying life without illness, mental or social disorder. (female)

A complete body/mental/social well-being. (gender not recorded)

Physical fitness, strength, suppleness, stamina linked with emotional, mental well-being and a social confidence. (female)

The concept of social wellbeing is interesting by reason of its rarity. The WHO definition of health (WHO, 1985) which relates to physical, social and emotional wellbeing has been used quite considerably in the literature and health education programmes. People have made reference to many aspects of social conditions in their definitions of health, but there were only four formal uses of the term 'social'.

Themes compared

When a more detailed look is taken of all health themes across all orga-nisations the following pattern emerges. In the major category of 'pre-vention', 10 people (30%, n = 33) felt that 'not to misuse or abuse oneself' was the most important thing that they could do. In the 'absence' category, 45 people (49%, n=91) felt that the 'absence of illness' was their basis for deciding what health meant to them. 'Presence' had two equal scores from 30 people (32%, n = 93); 30 people felt that 'wellbeing' reflected their understanding of health and 30 people felt that 'feeling good' summed up their understanding of health.

In the group who responded to 'ability', 46 people (37%, n = 123), listed 'ability to function/perform' as their basis for deciding on health. Of the group who responded to 'physical wellbeing', 165 people (53%, n = 309) used this broad title to describe health. The next highest group in this category was 'feeling fit' with 37 people (12%) responding.

The broad title of 'psychological wellbeing' was used by 112 people (84%, n = 134). In the group who listed 'spiritual wellbeing' themes, 22 people (29%, n = 75) listed 'enjoying life' as their way of describing health.

The comments made by people in relation to their understanding of the word health were tested against Kenney's (1992) article 'The consumer's views of health'. This was based on previous work on definitions of health. Kenney devised a questionnaire which contained twelve categories which have previously been used in definitions of health (Smith, 1981; Laffrey, 1986). These categories were used together with a Lickert scale to gain an understanding of people's concepts of health. An attempt was made to score the responses in this questionnaire to the twelve categories. This did not work. The difficulty arose because the responses in this questionnaire were formed by the respondents rather than scoring within a set range of items. Some of the responses were multifactored; it would have been possible to code or score these responses, but very few responses matched the items used by Kenney (1992). Kenney's categories were: 'Adaptation; clinical; role performance; body image; cognitive function; fitness; harmony; health promotion; positive mood; self-actualisation; self-concept; and social involvement'.

Models of health

If the quantitative measures of health are looked at (Figure 6.4), then the pattern or model that emerges is that of a mechanistic, structured model, a model that would not be inconsistent with a medical approach to health. The elements included in the model are the known and current measurements of ill health with additional features such as work and leisure effects. The latter two effects are often not included in the medical model. There is, however, an emerging interest in exercise within the medical model. Not the same attention is being given to the effects of work.

In this survey 92% of the people said they felt healthy; on many of the measures they scored a higher or more positive response than would be expected in the population generally. From this it could be inferred that people at work are healthier than the general population.

If the comments that people made are examined, there is still, in many cases, a use of language which related to the medical model, i.e. smoking, drinking, exercise, diet. There was also the use of other language which showed that some people saw health as wider than the medical or systemic model (Figure 6.5). For them, health included a sense of responsibility, a

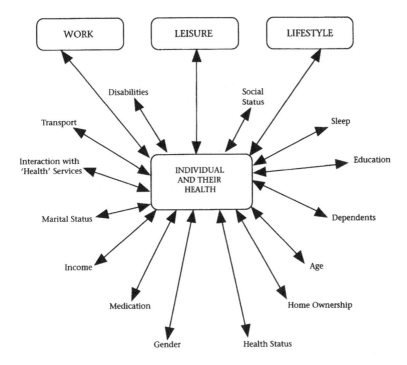

Figure 6.4   Influences on an individual and their health.

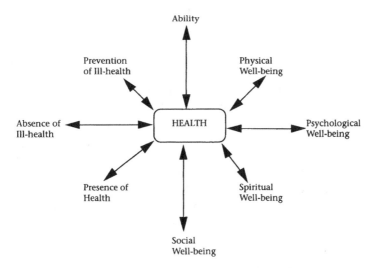

Figure 6.5   Perceptions of health.

responsibility to prevent ill health; a presence of health which they could articulate, an absence of ill health or disease which they knew made them healthy. For others, health was seen as physiological, physical function, physical imaging, physical responses.

For others, health is of the mind, of the soul, it is a feeling which they know, have felt, can describe. This second area of personal perceptions is

---

Case study : Mr X

Men can and do reflect on their health and the consequences of their actions on their health. Below is a case study produced from the questionnaire submitted by Mr X in the survey reported in this chapter (Bamford, 1993).

Mr X is 44 years old, working as an operator in a specialist metals organisation, which he has done for the last 16 years. He had done other jobs in the organisation, including packing and driving. He has worked in other organisations, having been a fireman on British Rail for eight years and a seaman for six years. Mr X now works 41 hours per week and does not now work shifts.

Mr X is married. His partner works, but he would not declare the joint income of the household, feeling that this was private. He left secondary modern school at or before 16 years old. He has dependent children, is an owner-occupier and has access to two cars.

Mr X feels he is not healthy and that his health is below average. His health history is:

0–1 years – did not regain birth weight for 14 weeks.
5–6 years – operation on left eye for lazy muscles.
10 years – removal of tonsils and adenoids.
17 years – road traffic accident: broke left femur, shattered patella, shattered os calcis, ruptured popliteal artery.
42 years – two heart attacks in 24 hours.
Now   – continuous pain from arthritis.

He feels that the health effects of leisure activities are good (he is an angler), work effects are bad, and the life he leads has had a good effect on his health. He has not seen his doctor in the past twelve months, and when he did see him it was because of his heart attack. Mr X feels that he has a permanent or long-standing illness, disability or infirmity as a result of his road traffic accident. He is not taking any medication. His hobbies include gardening and angling; he usually does his hobbies three or four times a week.

He has difficulty in getting to sleep, his mind is too active, and he has not slept properly since he finished working shifts $4\frac{1}{2}$ years ago. He is more the area which needs to be further explored. Some of the people in this survey who described themselves as healthy had medical or disease labels, some of them felt stressed, others had sleeping difficulties. Some described unhappiness, concern for their health, or personal behaviour which they knew was 'bad for their health'. Other people described their joy in living, their contentment, their happiness, their healthiness. The differences

---

concerned than worried about his health, and has felt worried and anxious about other things beside his health including all of the six categories – employment, money, family, relationships, well-being and 'other' – at various times.

He is a smoker, who is aware of the health effects of smoking and this understanding has affected how much he smokes. He drinks alcohol occasionally, considers alcohol's health effects to be poisonous, and this understanding has not affected his drinking habits.

Mr X has visited his occupational health department in the past twelve months; this was for a checkup on his heart condition. He has not been to see his GP, but was referred to hospital when he had his heart attack at work. He has felt ill during the past twelve months. He took time off work for one week with food poisoning.

For Mr X 'health' means:

Good or bad that's the question? Like it or not, health has become a commodity to be sold off. If left to what's left of the NHS there is just a slight chance that with the right care the patient may just get better.

He had some additional comments:

Started work age eight years in the Birmingham markets doing anything to support the family. I was working 16 hours a day on the railway with no set shift pattern. Work that made your hands blister through shovelling coal, your face ran with sweat and as you wiped it, the skin came off with the sweat. Your arms got sore because your jacket cut you and your legs ached because the engine went one way and the tender another. Your food was swilled down with coal dust, and you smoked your Woodbines in air that when the light caught it right would show you all the pretty colours in that dust. The railways made us redundant and we were sad. We should have thanked them.

Went deep sea fishing, saw boys become men overnight, worked three days at a stretch without a stand-down, them came the cod war and the rest is history, as they say.

Yes, my health is below average. I am an old man at 45 and no one cares because at the end of the day I will be just another faded photograph, and someone will say 'I remember him, What was his name?'.

between the two groups were not necessarily due to having a disease or medical condition. It was other factors, personal to an individual and within their own framework of positive or negative, good or bad, healthy or diseased, which people used to describe their perceptions of health.

This is the area where more work needs to be done, to identify the personal frameworks of individuals to see if there are commonalities. Do people in different organisational positions think differently about health; are they conditioned in relation to their expectations, the demands they expect to be placed on them, the rewards they expect to receive? It may be that people in this survey responded with the answers they felt were expected; it could be that in personal and private conversation a different, more personal model of health would emerge.

Effects of work, leisure and lifestyle on health

The effects of work on health have been reported on in more detail in Bamford (1993) and Bamford and Morton-Cooper (1997). In this chapter it needs to be noted that people have more negative views of the effects of work on health than the effects of leisure and lifestyle on health. The latter two activities are seen as being positive. In relation to the views about the positive and negative health effects of work there was a fairly equal distribution between men and women. People in this survey were asked if they had felt ill during the last twelve months, and out of 449 (98%) responses 275 (62%) had. This was 166 men (36%) and 109 (24%) women. When these people's responses were looked at in relation to their feelings of the effects of work the following distribution occurs: in all groups at least 50% of people had felt ill in the last 12 months, but in the fair–poor effect category, 77% of people had felt ill in the last twelve months.

When this group of people who had felt ill in the last twelve months are then looked at in relation to their views of their health average by gender, the following picture emerges. A total of 275 people (60%) who responded to the health average question had felt ill during the last 12 months. The highest proportion was in the group who felt their health was 'average' with 40% (184 people) feeling ill; this was the highest response for both men (116 – 42%) and women (68 – 25%).

Summary

In this chapter we have described some of the results of a major survey of the perceptions of their health of people at work. This shows much of the diversity of both men's and women's knowledge and attitudes. There are only a few topics where there are clear distinctions by gender. If the quotations did not have a male or female label attached to them, would you have been able to identify the gender? Do you feel that you should have known? Do we have preconceived views about how men and women articulate their views about health? The case study of Mr X shows how important it is to take a longitudinal perspective on the interaction between health and work.

We suggest in Chapter 9 how this study needs to be replicated and extended as part of the gendering of research on health and work.

Further reading

Bamford, M. (1993) *Aspects of health among an employed population*. Unpublished PhD. Thesis, Birmingham, Aston University.

Collinson, D. and Hearn, J. (1996) *Men as Managers. Managers as Men*. Sage, London.

Sennett, R. (1998) *The Corrosion of Character: the personal consequences of work in the new capitalism*. W.W. Norton & Co., London.

Chapter 7
National and International Perspectives

In this chapter we:

- suggest that health policy and services are not adequately gendered from the male perspective;
- discuss the need for a more strategic approach to addressing male health needs in England;
- describe strategic developments within the UK, including *The Health of the Nation* White Paper, *The New NHS* White Paper and *Our Healthier Nation* Green Paper, the Chief Medical Officer's 'Project to Strengthen the Public Health Function in England', and other national developments aimed at reducing health inequalities;
- describe international strategic case studies, including: the World Health Organisation's European Health For All Programme, European Commission public health policy, the Swiss Men's Health Charter and national and state activity in Australia;
- recommend ways forward at the strategic level, especially by introducing the two key perspectives – sex- and gender-specificity;
- highlight transferable ideas from Australia.

Introduction

The most important new conclusion that we have now reached is that something should be done about the health of men. (Professor R. Griffiths, Director of Public Health, former West Midlands Regional Health Authority, now National Health Executive West Midlands). (NHSE-WM, 1994, p. 118)

This chapter challenges the widely held, but little debated, assumption that health policy and services address the health needs of men in appropriate and effective ways. We assert instead that public health policy and programmes lack an adequately gendered perspective, i.e. one that takes a balanced view of the health needs of both sexes, rather than present activity which is more focused and holistic for female health needs but much more fragmented for male health needs. The result is that the NHS generally provides health services for males only in indirect and implicit ways.

This chapter, therefore, asks whether there should now be a strategy to address male health needs in explicit and direct ways. If the case can be made for such a strategic development, we ask what form should it take and at what levels. Should we argue for a distinct national male health policy or for an approach that seeks to integrate male perspectives into existing and new public health policy and programmes? Does it require central government or local health authorities to act, or maybe both?

The development of boys' and men's health policy and good practice is in its infancy, both internationally and nationally with considerable variation in progress across the industrialised world. This chapter describes and discusses case studies from within the UK, Europe and Australia (the country that has advanced the most in this field) and highlights opportunities for levering male health issues on the strategic agenda.

Earlier chapters have shown that the public health problem of boys' and men's health in this country is characterised by high levels of preventable premature mortality and avoidable ill health. Research for this chapter, therefore, concentrated on strategic activities which may address these issues across the whole population. Researching male health in this way is problematic for the following reasons: boys' and men's health has only recently been recognised as a problem; male-specific health services remain a very minor proportion of current NHS activity; and there has, so far, been only limited efforts nationally to facilitate networking among all active and interested parties.

The main sources of information used by Peter Williamson to research material for Chapters 7 and 8 were the existing local men's health networks and his own contacts in the field. These then often led to other useful contacts. Key individuals and departments within organisations and published and unpublished reports were the principal sources of information. Methods of communication included written correspondence, postal questionnaires, telephone interviews and e-mail.

As defined in Chapter 3, we use 'sex' to refer to the biological fact of male or female whereas 'gender' refers to the broader, sociological and cultural aspects of becoming and living as a boy and man, or girl and woman, in society today. 'Sex-specific', therefore, means uniquely relating to, or affecting, the biologically female or male. 'Gender-sensitive' means responsive to the different sociocultural aspects of being a male or female.

The chapter begins by debating the need for a male health strategy and describes the evolution of male health as a major health issue. It then gives some background to the development of recent health strategy for England: The Health of the Nation (HoN) strategy; and its successor Our Healthier Nation (OHN) strategy. At the time of writing (June 1999), the OHN

Green Paper consultation document has not yet been replaced by the long promised White Paper. Two responses to OHN from men's health groups are outlined.

We then explore how two recent initiatives about health inequalities approach the topic of sex inequalities. These are the 'Independent Inquiry into Inequalities in Health' and the Economic and Social Research Council's research programme on 'Variations in Health'.

The most important health services policy development of the Labour government is the White Paper *The New NHS*. We examine the implications for male health of health improvement programmes, primary care groups, and the national performance framework. A second development, which has considerable potential, is the Chief Medical Officer's Project to Strengthen the Public Health Function in England which emphasises the need to involve the public and encourage local projects. Both of these developments could benefit male health.

Health policy of international agencies, such as the World Health Organization's European Health For All Programme and its sponsorship and support for the Healthy Cities projects, and the European Community's public health programme are described and evaluated with regard to male health.

The country which has paid most attention to male health is Australia, and the chapter ends with detailed reviews of the federal and two states' policies. These case studies provide useful examples of what male health policies look like, and there are also lessons to learn about the difficulties of policy development, the perils of 'going public' and encountering political backlash.

The need for strategic development

In the NHS, and in other areas of the public sector, males appear not to have been perceived historically as a specific population group when services are planned and delivered: in general, this has remained the status quo. Gender (here meaning sex) was only recently officially recognised as a significant factor affecting inequalities in health in the UK. In the public health sphere, it seems that there is a reluctance to consider health needs from the sex point of view. Since the Black report (Townsend and Davidson, 1982), social class has remained the key stratification variable in health policy. Other variables such as sex, ethnicity and age are often seen as less important.

Since the *Health of the Nation* strategy, and perhaps for some time before then, sex-specific public health and health promotion programmes targeting males have not been implemented in the same way as those for females. At the population level, there are good reasons for this and it is over simplistic to argue for a more equitable provision of, for example, screening services for males. As Worth writes:

> This sex-specific approach encourages comparisons with the women's health movement: campaigns for national screening programmes for prostatic and testicular cancer appear similar to the screening programme for breast cancer. Such an approach may have its place. (Worth, 1997, p. 12)

The major exception among males are HIV prevention programmes among gay and bisexual men across the whole population. Such programmes have been part of mainstream preventive health service activity since the mid-1980s. However, this exception highlights the lack of programmes that directly target males to prevent other major public health problems, e.g. heart disease and stroke, cancer of the lung, bowel or skin, suicide and accidents. Of course, there are population-based preventive programmes for most of these health problems, but males are seldom explicitly targeted as a priority group.

Furthermore, the perspective on gender within health, social and educational studies has usually been women-centred. There is a need, as the 21st century approaches, to redress the balance of attentions paid towards male health issues when considering gender and health.

> Among the outcomes of a heightened social awareness of issues of equal opportunities, policy makers have for the past few years given increased attention to women's health; men's health, on the other hand, has received less emphasis. (Worth, 1997, p. 11)

Health research often assumes that males are a homogenous group representing the norm against which other social groups can be compared and defined as 'abnormal', i.e. possessing different and sometimes more important needs. However, males often predominantly appear as members of those social groups that are defined and labelled as having more significant needs, e.g. young people, the unemployed, working class, black, gay and bisexual, disabled, and mentally ill. Stratification, such as socio-economic status, ethnicity, sexual identity and age, have been considered to exert greater influence than that of sex and gender.

The male population has been lumped together as an amorphous mass. When diversity is recognised, males are judged apart from each other by comparison with the dominant social group. The dominant type of man is the one that is more likely to be socially approved of and that tends to hold most power over others: white, employed, heterosexual and married, ablebodied, middle class and mentally well. These values permeate health services.

> ... the dominant white, heterosexual male, order has become seen as the natural order against which 'others' are measured ... the sexual division of

labour [in health services] has led to higher values being attached to 'male' roles (medicine) and lower values attached to 'female' roles (nursing) ... this process has [also] created the gendered structure seen in the NHS leading to an organisation built on, and valuing, the 'masculine' stereotypes of strength, rationality and productivity over the 'feminine' contribution of care, nurturing and subjectivity ... this structure was strengthened by the 'new right' ideologies of the mid-1990s, the belief in competition via the internal market which produced a business culture in the NHS. (Robertson, 1998, p. 47)

Government health and social policy

National developments

The Conservative government produced *The Health of the Nation* White Paper in 1992 which became the UK's first national health strategy. The Labour government has now produced the Green Paper for the second strategy for England, *Our Healthier Nation.*

Sir Donald Acheson briefly highlighted male health needs towards the end of his term of office as Chief Medical Officer (CMO) for England in the early 1990s. The health needs of males as a population group were documented officially and more comprehensively for the first time in 1993 through the dedication of a whole chapter to the subject by the then Chief Medical Officer, Sir Kenneth Calman, in his annual report for 1992. He concluded by stating: 'It is hoped that Regions and Districts will investigate ways to promote the health of men over the next few years' (DOH, 1993).

Since the launch of the first health strategy for England, and despite this recognition by the CMO, there has been no substantive leadership, direction or co-ordination of efforts within government to address the major and historical public health problem of male health across the country. There have, however, been some significant developments within government, including some financial investment, which could have benefits.

Under the last Conservative administration, the CMO's Health of the Nation Working Group set up the Variations in Health subgroup, which was charged to review the available evidence and recommend what the Department of Health and the NHS could do to reduce existing variations. The subgroup's report, published in 1995, recognised gender (here meaning sex) as one of a number of key variables influencing health variations together with social class, age, ethnicity and region of residence.

One of this report's recommendations was to conduct more research. In 1997, the Economic and Social Research Council launched its Health Variations Research Programme based at the University of Lancaster and directed by Professor Hilary Graham. Phase one involves 13 major research studies being performed by accredited research units and university departments across the UK. Phase two was expected to launch another set of research projects at the end of last year (Graham, 1998a).

At a more operational level, the National Health Service Executive (NHSE) has issued guidance to health authorities emphasising the importance of equity, which it described as improving the health of the population as a whole and: 'reducing variations in health status by targeting resources where needs are greatest' (NHSE, 1995).

Health authorities were asked:

> to pay particular attention to variations in health status when planning how to use resources directly available to them, and through collaborating with others. (DOH , 1997a)

Performance management frameworks, brought in to monitor progress towards meeting the Health of the Nation objectives, included reference to the needs of vulnerable population groups. These have now been superseded by a new national performance framework under the Labour government.

In its efforts to adopt a more positive approach to male health, in general, the Department of Health set up an internal Men's Health Team in 1993 as a consequence of the chapter dedicated to the health of men in the CMO's annual report for 1992. This appears to have been an administrative development with the team focusing on health promotion and liaison with other units and teams engaged in work relevant to men, e.g. AIDS and circumcision. Its main achievement was the production of the first general health information leaflet for men at the national level, *Life begins at 40 – health tips for men*. It appears that the team disbanded following the publicity campaign that launched the leaflet in May 1998. There has been no evaluation of the impact of this campaign.

In the mid-1990s, the Department of Health funded three men's health promotion research projects through small grants. These are:

- *Men's Health: Ducking the Targets?*: a programme to identify how to enable men to take up health promotion messages and opportunities more effectively. This was managed by Community Health UK, the national community health development charity. This programme was initially funded for 18 months, but no report has ever been published.
- *Alive and Kicking*: a project managed by the Community Education and Development Centre in Coventry. An evaluation report was published (CEDC, 1997). Further DOH funding has allowed a second project to begin in Nuneaton, Coventry and Warrington.
- *The Nu Black Initiative*: a project to promote health awareness among black men managed by the West Indian Standing Conference.

At the international level, in 1995, the UK government signed a United Nations (UN) resolution to 'mainstream a gender perspective into all policies and programmes'. This took place at the Fourth UN World Conference on Women in Beijing, China. The NHS Executive took on responsibility to implement this policy in the health sector and, in the following year, held a national conference, 'Making Gender Matter in Health Care and Health Promotion'. No report was ever published of this conference, but it is reported to have:

> explored the importance of 'gender perspectives' with NHS purchasers and providers of health care, and considered cost-effective ways to make health services more sensitive to the differing needs of men and women. (DOH, 1997a)

In the intervening period until the 1997 general election, government undertook no further work on this policy directive regarding the health of males, although this has not been the case in the women's policy field. It appears that the 1995 NHS conference on gender and health marked the end of central activity and that health authorities are now expected to take things further. The Department of Health did announce, however, the previously mentioned new male health publicity programme targeting 40–69-year-olds which was to have been launched in 1997. Unfortunately, the general election delayed the campaign launch until May 1998.

Following the 1997 general election, the incoming Labour government set up another major investigation into variations in health. Part of the remit of the Independent Inquiry into Inequalities in Health, chaired by former CMO, Sir Donald Acheson, was to identify, in the light of a review of the evidence:

> ... priority areas for future policy development ... likely to offer opportunities for Government to develop beneficial, cost effective and affordable interventions to reduce health inequalities. (Acheson, 1998)

The Report was published in late 1998. Its findings are to be integrated into the process of drawing up the new health strategy.

Whilst these steps are not directed solely at addressing male health needs, they represent a more explicit recognition of sex differences in health. Apart from the previously mentioned conferences in 1994 and 1996, the only other major development with the potential for influencing national health strategy as it affects males was the establishment by the Royal College of Nursing of the Men's Health Forum in 1994 (discussed in Chapter 8). This came in response to a motion passed by delegates at their annual congress.

The Health of the Nation strategy

The Health of the Nation White Paper was the first time that England had had a national health strategy. Therefore, the way in which the strategy was formulated and implemented had important implications for male health. The lessons learnt will be discussed further in Chapter 9.

By identifying the five key areas for action, the government opted for a disease-led approach. Individual responsibility for health was emphasised at the expense of an acknowledgement of a sociocultural dimension of health. It was felt that the government did not want to refer to poverty as a factor. However, the government claimed that:

> the phrase, 'men's health', has tended to feel unfamiliar ... [yet] there's no good refusing to concentrate on the particular themes of health that apply to men. We're so used to hearing about women's health, child health etc., it has tended to be accepted that there were things which we could learn by looking specifically at the diseases, behaviours and attitudes associated with women and children and targeting our approaches accordingly. But, ... having said that, men haven't been neglected. Enormous resources have always gone into researching and treating those diseases, such as heart disease and lung cancer, which affect men disproportionately. Likewise, health promotion has always focused on the sort of risky behaviour practised by some men and on the potential for reducing the burden of avoidable illness and early death. Perhaps, though, it has taken a little longer to recognise that, just as with women and children, there may be some new and added insights for us in looking at men as a population group, when planning strategies to prevent and treat ill-health.
>
> Health of the Nation [HoN] is ..., in one sense, a strategy to improve the health of men. It is not just that some of the targets are specific to men. HoN focuses ... attention ... on the high rates of coronary disease in men, the way in which lung cancer is especially prevalent in men, the high suicide rates for men in the 15–34 year age group, on sexual and drug using behaviour, which puts men at risk of HIV infection and on accidents, where young men are four times more likely than young women to be involved. For the first time, the health status of men is put in clear focus and the HoN strategy gives us the vehicle to do something about it. (Tom Sackville, MP for Bolton West, Under Secretary of State for Health, Conservative government 1995) (Sackville, 1995)

At the local level, opportunities were seen by some health authorities to incorporate male health in the five key areas:

> several of the Health of the Nation targets relate very closely to male health issues, [and] services will need specifically to address these so that targets may be met. (Worth, 1997)

Others were not so clear:

> My problem remains that I still have no clear idea of what we should do, rather than why. A large part of Health of the Nation is directed towards men, if you

> look at the relative rates of illness for men and women. I can see that different
> approaches might be needed for men and women... I feel as if I am colour-
> blind or tone deaf and missing something very obvious to others – but I am
> missing it. (Anonymous communication)

There is very little evidence of government following up its 1995 commitment to mainstream gender into all policies and programmes with any
concrete action regarding male health.

Our Healthier Nation strategy

One of the early actions with respect to health policy by the incoming
Labour government in 1997 was the Green Paper *Our Healthier Nation*. It
was intended to make a major revision to the national health strategy.
Whilst it did not completely move away from a focus on conditions – it
identified four priority areas – poverty and its relationship to inequalities in
health in society have been given centre stage.

> we do not have specific policies aimed at men *per se*, although of course,
> much of our cardiovascular disease prevention work is *implicitly* [author's
> emphasis] aimed at men.... I believe that the health of men is something that
> has been overlooked. It is time that we recognised that men have shorter lives,
> suffer in excess of many illnesses, and often have less good emotional and
> support networks than their female counterparts. (Woodhouse, 1998)

Analysing the consultation responses

The request for consultation on the Green Paper, *Our Healthier Nation*
offered an opportunity for those interested in male health to make an
impact. The way in which responses were handled is of interest for future
attempts to influence policy making in central government, which will be
taken up in Chapter 9. The Health Strategy Unit at the Department of
Health was responsible for handling responses to the Green Paper *Our
Healthier Nation*. Initially, all responses were read through to identify the
issues they raised against a list of about 50 'key words'. Depending on the
key issues in a response, all responses were then copied, as appropriate, to
departmental staff (key leads) with responsibility for particular issues for
greater analysis.

Sex differences in health were designated to be part of the investigation
carried out by the Independent Inquiry into Inequalities in Health. For this
reason, *neither men's or male health nor gender were selected as key words
for the initial analysis of responses to the Green Paper*. All responses which
raised issues that could be categorised under the wider key word heading of

'health inequalities' were copied to the support team for Independent Inquiry into Inequalities in Health. During the research period for this chapter, it was, therefore, not possible to obtain comprehensive information about the number of male health responses submitted (with male health as the only theme or one of several) and the number and nature of the agencies or organisations that submitted them. However, the Department of Health was able to indicate that three responses were received from organisations with men's health in their titles: the East Midlands Men's Health Network; the Men's Health Forum; and, the Men's Health Trust. The first two responses are summarised below.

Unfortunately, it was also not possible to get a sense of the individual or collective impact of any male health responses to the Green Paper for the same reason. Findings from Independent Inquiry into Inequalities in Health are expected to be fed directly into the forthcoming White Paper *Our Healthier Nation*.

Response from the East Midlands Men's Health Network

There is a relative lack of recognition of the influence of both the variables of sex (biology) and of gender (culture) compared to that of social class on inequalities in health. There is inadequate recognition, and no consequent attempt at prioritisation of the relative importance of, documented significant sex differences in health. Finally, there is inadequate recognition of the complex inter-relationships between social class, age, sex, gender, race and their effects on health (Williamson and Jackson, 1998).

In addition to these points Williamson and Jackson (1998) consider that there is a lack of analytical commentary on the influence of the variables of sex and gender attached to the reports, and diagrammatic presentations, of statistics on men and women.

This omission is not helped by the fact that there is a systematic under-reporting of male health needs. There is a specific lack of an informed understanding of how gender, masculinity (i.e. how males see themselves as boys and men in our society) and power directly affect the health state and experience of males.

For these reasons, there is a need to fund more public health research in order to build a sound evidence base to shape men's health policy and practice. The following points must be addressed.

- Research, especially of a qualitative nature, is required into the health of males as a population group and into the different experiences of the diverse groups of boys and men in our society, e.g. older, gay and bisexual, working class, unemployed, disabled, Asian and Afro-Caribbean.

- More precise targeting is required of social factors known to have an influence on male health, e.g. on health-damaging behaviours and environments.
- There is a need for more piloting of public health interventions, e.g. preventive programmes, that address male health issues.
- The knowledge gathered through the above research activity must play a part in informing the policy-making process.
- In order to conduct sound research, policy and practice, there is a need to build alliances between key agencies to address the health needs of males.
- There is a need to identify effective ways of involving the local male population.
- There is a need to address the specific needs of boys and girls in the setting of schools (Making Healthy Schools should become a reality for boys).
- There is a need to develop evidence-based practice on gender issues affecting boys.

Response from the Men's Health Forum

The following key points were made in the submission (Banks and Mason, 1998):

- Gender inequalities, which form a major contributory factor in health variations, are not placed as highly as might be considered appropriate. Given clear gender inequalities, there remains scope for more clearly defining targets.
- The Green Paper recognises that health inequalities exist between men and women, including in the target areas. However, the different health experiences of men are not reflected in the targets.
- More work is needed in assessing and monitoring access to, and take-up of, health information by men.
- Demonstration projects in this area should be an early innovation.

Government social exclusion policy

Further insight into the direction of public policy can be gained through a brief consideration of how government intends to address the problems of social exclusion. Social exclusion is defined as:

> a shorthand label for what can happen when individuals or areas suffer from a combination of linked problems such as unemployment, poor skills, low incomes, poor housing, high crime environments, bad health and family breakdown. (SEU, 1997)

Social exclusion policy has direct relevance to public health. Firstly, there are important health consequences to communities experiencing such problems. Secondly, the stated direction of both health and social exclusion policies is towards reducing inequalities in society. Key questions, therefore, are to what extent does social exclusion affect the sexes differently and how much of this difference does government recognise, and, in this context, in relation to boys and men, in particular?

The Prime Minister launched the Social Exclusion Unit (SEU), part of the Economic and Domestic Affairs Secretariat in the Cabinet Office, in a speech in December 1997. In his first prime ministerial speech six months earlier, made to announce the new government's broad agenda for society, he trailed social exclusion as a government priority. Although there is no specific reference to sex and gender in the former speech, there is in the latter in relation to unemployment and family breakdown, when he states:

> For a generation of young men, little has come to replace the third of all manufacturing jobs that have been lost. For part of a generation of young women early pregnancies and the absence of a reliable father almost guarantee a life of poverty, and today Britain has a higher proportion of single parent families than anywhere else in Europe. (Blair, 1997)

The SEU was set up to reduce social exclusion by arriving at a better understanding of the issue and of how government policy impacts on it and by co-ordinating and improving action across government. Initial priority areas have included truancy and social exclusion, street living and rough sleeping, sink housing estates, teenage parenthood and 16- to 18-year-olds not in education, training or employment.

Truancy and school exclusion

According to the SEU, there is no sex bias in the prevalence of, and trends over time in, truancy, but most excluded pupils are male, white, young teenagers. The unit quantifies these problems by stating that:

> each year at least one million children truant, and over 100 000 children are excluded temporarily. Some 13 000 are excluded permanently. (SEU, 1998a)

and qualifies the longer term impact of the problems on individuals by continuing:

> both truancy and exclusion are associated with a significantly higher likelihood of becoming a teenage parent, being unemployed or homeless later in life, or ending up in prison. (SEU, 1998a)

The major impact on the wider community is identified as the resultant high level of criminal activity.

Sleeping rough

The SEU reports that:

> Over the course of a year, at least 2400 people spend some time sleeping
> rough in London. 1800 are new arrivals. . . . The total on any given night . . .
> averages about 400. . . . It is estimated that in England perhaps 2000 sleep
> rough each night which probably means 10 000 drift in and out of rough
> sleeping over the course of a year. (SEU, 1998b)

Although information on the backgrounds of people sleeping rough is
limited, it is the most highly gendered of the SEU's priority areas in terms of
the population it directly affects: about 90% of rough sleepers are male.

A link is apparent between rough sleepers and a major cause of premature mortality among men in that:

> a study of Coroners' courts found that death by unnatural causes for rough
> sleepers was four times more common than average and suicide thirty-five
> times more likely. (SEU, 1998b)

Teenage parenthood

Whilst this issue is obviously gendered from the female perspective, there
are important implications for male teenagers in relation to unsafe sex and
unintended pregnancy. There are two references to boys and men in consultation questions. One asks: 'Do you think boys and girls should be taught
together or separately?' (SEU, 1998c). The other asks: 'What should be
expected of young fathers and how could they be helped to make their
contribution?' (SEU, 1998c)

Conclusion

The Labour government repeatedly describes social exclusion as a set of
joined up problems requiring joined up solutions. Yet it has only partially
grasped the fact that many of the main features of the nature of some social
exclusion problems and, by implication, of solutions to them are clearly
gendered from the male dimension. The link is that where males represent
the majority of those directly affected, masculinities (i.e. ways of being a
boy and living and working as a man in contemporary society) are highly
likely to be related to both the problem and to how best to tackle it.

By not clearly acknowledging this perspective, neither gender in general,
nor boys and men in particular are directly named up front. Thus, for
example, the Department of Health proposed to sponsor:

[a] research project to identify areas where rough sleepers and homeless people are having persistent problems gaining access to GPs. (SEU, 1998b)

This presents an opportunity of linking this access to health care issue for rough sleepers up with the lower GP consultation rate among men, as a whole, when compared with women.

Disappointingly, there is very little evidence from the work of the Social Exclusion Unit that the Labour government has chosen to abide by the commitment to integrate a gender perspective into all mainstream policies and programmes (especially from a male perspective) made by the previous Conservative administration.

The Independent Inquiry into Inequalities in Health

In total, the inquiry received approximately 300 contributions of solicited and unsolicited evidence. As well as considering this evidence, a series of presentations was made to the inquiry on a number of relevant issues.

Only a small number of submissions solely addressed sex and gender issues. However, sex and gender were covered by a significant proportion of submissions on a range of other issues. It was decided not to analyse evidence to the inquiry by subject area, partly due to the difficulty of trawling through so many contributions.

A section of the inquiry's report addresses sex and socio-economic differences in general causes of mortality and morbidity:

the approach of the Inquiry has been to focus on gender and socioeconomic health differences in terms of mortality and morbidity from general rather than gender specific causes. The Inquiry has noted the higher incidence of mortality in men than women at every age. Mortality in young men is of particular concern, not least because of the years of life lost. (Earwicker, 1998)

Moreover, as reference is made to sex differences in other parts of the report, the sections on adults and on employment also mention issues that affect young men in particular.

Research into health inequalities

There has been a recent rekindling of public health research into health inequalities in the light of a changed political environment more sympathetic to the issue. As Professor Hilary Graham of the Economic and Social Research Council's (ESRC) research programme states: 'Tackling health inequalities is at the heart of the public health strategy of the Labour government' (Graham, 1998a).

The Economic and Social Research Council's Health Variations Programme

The establishment of the Variations in Health Research Programme funded by the Economic and Social Research Council, based at the University of Lancaster, in part reflects the change in government attention paid to health inequalities after the transition from the Conservative to Labour government. The Thatcher-led Conservative government had refused to recognise either the links between poverty and poorer health or the existence of health inequalities. Whilst the Major government took a similar line on poverty, it did begin to talk about variations in health, its preferred term for health inequalities.

At the Department of Health, the then Chief Medical Officer for England, Sir Kenneth Calman, established a Variations Sub-Group of his Health of the Nation Working Group:

> to advise on what the Department of Health and the NHS could do to tackle ethnic, geographical, socio-economic and *gender* [author's emphasis] variations in health within the key areas identified by the Health of the Nation. . . . These variations are associated with a range of often interacting factors: geography, socio-economic status, *gender* [author's emphasis], environment, ethnicity, culture, and lifestyle. (NHS Executive, 1995)

This development not only reawakened official government recognition of the existence of health inequalities absent since Margaret Thatcher came to power in 1979, but it also represented official government acknowledgement of the importance of sex differences within health inequalities. It appears, however, that 'gender' in the above quotes actually refers to sex and not to the wider definition of gender used in this book.

In their report, the sub-group outlined the NHS's responsibilities for acting on variations in health and made recommendations for action by the NHS and the Department of Health. These have now been superseded by the Green Paper *Our Healthier Nation*.

A specific outcome of the sub-group's work was that, in 1996, the Department of Health then commissioned a £2.4 million research initiative. This became the ESRC's research programme on health variations that:

> aims to advance understanding of the social factors which underlie socio-economic differences in health in ways which contribute to the development of strategies which narrow the health gap between socio-economic groups . . . [e.g.] gender differences: how does the socio-economic patterning of health vary between men and women? (Graham, 1998a)

The research programme, therefore, concentrates on socio-economic or class differences in health and the processes that produce them. Factors, like sex, age and ethnicity, are not the focus of the programme, but as they all contribute to these processes, they will be inherent in all studies' analyses (Graham, 1998b).

Phase one consisted of 13 studies. Of these, three not only include sex in their analysis but also take some account of gender.

The Role of Perceptions of Family History in Persisting Inequalities in Health and Lifestyles (University of Glasgow)

This study (ESRC, 1997) sets out to explore how perceptions of having a family history of heart disease might influence health-related behaviours (such as smoking, diet and consumption of alcohol). Women have lower rates of coronary heart disease than men, and they are often assumed to be the guardians of their families' health. This study will compare the experience of family history of heart disease in men and women of different social classes in relation to individual perceptions of familial susceptibility to major chronic illness and how each effects current coronary health promotion. (ESRC,1998, p. 9)

Social Settings at Home and Work: Early and Later Life Influences on Health Variations (Institute of Child Health)

... This piece of research set out to examine the extent to which adult life experiences in the home or work environment (such as social support, and job strain and insecurity) and early life factors contribute towards the development of health inequalities, and whether these influences affect men and women in similar ways. (ESRC, 1998, pp. 14–15)

Ethnic Variations in Health: Assessing the Role of Class, Gender and Geography (Policy Studies Institute)

The third piece of work was undertaken 'to assess the importance of socio-economic status, gender and geography in ethnic variations in health'. (ESRC, 1998, p. 9)

In conclusion, the ESRC's Health Variations Research Programme not only recognises the importance of sex differences, it also explicitly acknowledges the potential influence or role of gender:

our gender is of fundamental importance in determining the course of our lives. Understanding how our gendered biographies may protect us from some aspects of ill-health but predispose us to others is ... important for understanding the relationship between gender and health. (ESRC, 1998, p. 9)

Extending research into health inequalities beyond its previously limited focus on sex to one that also encompasses gender will contribute to a fuller understanding of the causes of male health inequalities and how best to tackle them.

The New NHS – Modern and Dependable

This White Paper (DOH, 1997b), published in December 1997, included at least three important new developments for the NHS that present leverage opportunities for male health at the strategic level both locally and nationally:

- Health Improvement Programmes;
- Primary Care Groups;
- a national performance framework for NHS services.

Health Improvement Programmes

A Health Improvement Programme (HImP) is defined as:

> An action programme led by the Health Authority to improve health and health care locally [that] will involve NHS Trusts, Primary Care Groups and other primary care professionals, working in partnership with the local authority and other local interests. (DOH, 1997b, p. 13)

The Labour government expects that HImPs will serve to redress the fragmentation, as the Labour Party saw it when in opposition, of the planning and delivery of health and social care services to patients.

Health authorities were required to have their first HImPs in place by April 1999. Under the previous government's strategy *Health of the Nation*, health authority purchasing plans were required every year. HImPs will cover a three year period allowing for annual reviews. Amongst other proposed features of a HImP are that they will:

> set out a range of locally-determined priorities and targets to address issues and problems which are judged important, with particular emphasis on addressing areas of major health inequality in local communities; (DOH, 1998a, p. 40)

> show that the action proposed is based on evidence of what is known to work (from research and best practice reports). (DOH, 1998a, p. 41)

Primary Care Groups

The Labour government also introduced Primary Care Groups (PCGs) via *The New NHS* White Paper in its efforts to develop the commissioning of local health services beyond GP fundholding. The White Paper states that: 'the Government wants to keep what has worked about fundholding, but discard what has not' (DOH, 1997b, p. 33).

It continues:

> The Government therefore intends to establish Primary Care Groups across the country, bringing together GPs and community nurses in each area to work together to improve the health of local people. Primary Care Groups will grow out of a range of commissioning models that have developed in recent years but will give a sharper focus to their work. (DOH, 1997b, pp. 33–4)

PCGs will serve about 100 000 people, will bring together a number of GP practices already providing a service within the area lived in by that population and were expected to have agreed boundaries and established themselves by April 1999. Amongst other proposed main functions of PCGs are:

- to contribute to the Health Authority's Health Improvement Programme on health and health care, helping to ensure that this reflects the perspective of the local community and the experience of patients;
- to promote the health of the local population, working in partnership with other local agencies;
- to commission health services for their populations ... within the framework of the HImP, ensuring quality and efficiency;
- to monitor performance against ... service agreements;
- to develop primary care by joint working across practices;
- to better integrate primary and community health services (DOH, 1997b, p. 34)

A new national performance framework

The Labour government introduced a new national performance framework from April 1999 that replaces the previous government's NHS measurement tools, such as the Purchaser Efficiency Index.

> There must be improvements in quality and efficiency. Improvements in speed of access to care. Improvements to health, tackling past inequalities. ... The new framework will demonstrate progress on the overall goals of the NHS, on the key steps the NHS must take to deliver those goals, and on the outcomes it is achieving. (DOH, 1997b, pp. 63–4)

Of the six dimensions to the performance framework, three are particularly relevant to male health needs:

- *Health improvement*: to reflect the overall aim of improving the general health of the population ... for example, changes in rates of premature death, reflecting social and economic factors as well as health care.

- *Fair access*: to recognise that the NHS contribution must begin by offering fair access to health services in relation to people's needs irrespective of geography, class, ethnicity, age or sex.
- *Effective delivery of appropriate health care*: to recognise that fair access must be to care that is effective, appropriate and timely, and complies with agreed standards. (DOH, 1997b, p. 64)

Not only can NHS progress towards reducing the overarching male inequality in life expectancy be monitored, but also its progress towards addressing the male inequalities in:

- mortality rates in all age groups from birth to death;
- certain cause-specific death rates, particularly in relation to heart disease, lung and other cancers, accidents and suicide in different age groups;
- certain health-related behaviours, such as alcohol consumption, illicit drug use, sexual activity, healthy eating and other risk-taking behaviours, e.g. car driving;
- uptake of primary and community health services, including delayed help-seeking and resistance to taking health promotion opportunities up and messages on board.

The dimension of effective health care delivery can be extended to include public health and health promotion initiatives targeting males and ties in with the issue of the lack of evidence-based information on such schemes that was raised above in response to the *Our Healthier Nation* Green Paper.

The opportunities to advocate for action to address male health needs locally, presented by HImPs and PCGs, and centrally, by the national NHS performance framework, can be complemented by opportunities for advocacy on the development the government's proposed national contract for health.

> The contract sets out our mutual responsibilities for improving health in areas where we can make most progress towards our overall aims of reducing the number of early deaths, increasing the health of our healthy lives and tackling inequalities in health. (DOH, 1998a, p. 29)

The national contract stipulates the part to be played by government and other national players, communities and other local players, and individual people. A contract is proposed for each of the four national priority areas and related targets. Two key themes should run through the development and implementation of the national contract for health, HImPs and the national performance framework: sex-specificity and gender-sensitivity. Sex-specificity would ensure that significant sex differences in health at the population level are recognised and acted upon. Gender-sensitivity would ensure that the impact of sociocultural factors (as opposed to only biological aspects) of being male or female are also assessed and included. This could be one way of turning the government's commitment to reduce health inequalities into specific action regarding variations between males and females. It would also facilitate the transfer of a male dimension through to local strategic planning via the HImP.

The review of the public health function

In summer 1997, the Chief Medical Officer was asked by ministers to

lead a project to consider the range of current public health activities at local, regional and national levels, with a view to ensuring that there is a robust public health function to deliver the government's public health agenda. (DOH, 1998b, p. 1)

In February 1998, an interim report stated that the project:

has considered the public health function in its widest sense and not just the contribution made by public health professionals. It covers the vital role of many agencies such as local government, voluntary organisations, universities and others as well as the NHS. (DOH, 1998b, p. 1)

This emphasis on multi-agency collaboration echoes a main principle of the approach this chapter recommends in order to address male health needs at the strategic level.

A final report was expected in the autumn of 1998. Its findings would be relevant to both *The New NHS* White Paper and to the *Our Healthier Nation* White Paper (not published at the time of writing, June 1999).

The interim report identified five major themes involved in strengthening the public health function, all of which are relevant when considering how to promote male health:

- a wider understanding of health:

    a shared understanding of what can be done to improve population health, and of how people and organisations can contribute. Research to improve the evidence base for public health action, and better information about health, are essential components. (DOH, 1998b, p. 4);

- better co-ordination;
- an increase in capacity and capabilities;
- sustained development;
- effective joint working.

The report goes on to identify short- and medium-term action plans for public involvement, local and community, regional and national action and for research and development. Many of the action points require a gendered perspective to take account of their implications for promoting male health.

Involving the public

Recommended action includes engaging the public in a dialogue about HImPs, Health Action Zones and Healthy Living Centres and producing local and national strategies to involve the public in health matters. In the medium term, evidence of effective public involvement and developing good practice are called for. For this action to be applied to males, there is a need for research into, and development of, models for how to reach and involve boys and men locally and in a meaningful way.

Medium-term action makes particular mention of harder to reach groups of people, as there is a need to:

> actively promote the participation of those least likely to be involved and in greatest need because of social exclusion, vulnerability or existing poor health. (DOH, 1998b, p. 9)

This has a particular application to certain groups of men, as does the reported need to: provide education for health and active citizenship in schools, youth and adult education and training settings (DOH, 1998b, p. 9).

Investing in active citizenship through such settings will contribute towards greater social capital and cohesion among individual males.

The local and community level

> It is at the local level that public involvement through community action can be powerful ... shared populations of interest ... natural communities. (DOH, 1998b, p. 9)

It is important to ask the gendered question: *What does 'community' mean to different groups of boys and men?* Outreach and community development methods are proposed. What is the evidence of effectiveness of such methods to reach and engage different groups of men?

In light of the recommendation that PCGs should have a clear role to promote the health of their local community, they will require adequate public health capacity to:

- examine health and illness data on males and females from existing information sources situated at GP practice, health locality or health authority level in order to identify significant sex differences in their population and to identify gaps in available information;

- seek ways of consulting males about their health and how to improve it in order to fill the identified information gap.

A collaborative approach is recommended locally and this is particularly important with regard to improving male population health, as:

- primary health care services could benefit from joint working with local education and welfare services, who have traditionally had more experience of directly working with larger numbers of boys and men;
- if PCGs are to make an effective contribution, they will need to consider how neighbouring GP practices can work with each other and across their patient lists in order to reach males in appropriate contexts.

The regional level

[the regions need to] play a lead role in developing public health intelligence and disseminating information; ... [to] promote amongst the public, professionals and organisations wider understanding of health and ill-health and how these can be tackled. (DOH, 1998b, p. 15)

This requires the regional public heath function to pay attention to sex-specificity and gender-sensitivity as key themes. Significant sex differences in health must be made explicit, as do the relative influence of sociocultural factors on health status, for both men and women.

Research and development

Research in a wide range of disciplines is relevant to public health. A more co-ordinated approach to setting priorities for research, which contributes to improving the public's health, should be pursued. Long term research is needed to build the evidence base for public health improvement. (DOH, 1998b, p. 19)

This recommendation could equally apply to male health. A multi-disciplinary knowledge base is required. A research agenda is needed, on the one hand, to put sex differences in health in a priority list alongside other health inequalities and, on the other, to distinguish significant male from female health needs. *No evidence base as yet exists for effective male health improvement.*

The second recommendation is equally relevant to men's health.

A range of methodology is appropriate for public health research and it is not always straightforward to obtain funding for qualitative approaches. A particular area highlighted as problematic is research to evaluate local approaches to changing the public's health and the dissemination of such results to develop and share good practice. (DOH, 1998b, p. 19)

At health authority level, local research and development strategy should explore through qualitative research on social factors, such as:

employment and whether the expectations attached to their [men's] social role are met … [and] … Loss of employment and diminution of the male role. (Worth, 1997, p. 12)

Worth continues:

It is increasingly important that the Health Authority remains alert to and tries to act on research findings which have a particular relevance to men and their health (p. 17)

due to the fact that:

there is little evidence of effective interventions to remedy the inequalities in health faced by men. The experience of the HIV/AIDS programmes suggests that men need to be targeted, particularly at places where they meet together. Even though equal opportunities for all men to enjoy good health could ultimately only be achieved only by redressing social inequalities, more can certainly be done to make health care more accessible and to promote good health, especially in the workplace (p. 17).

Qualitative research on health-related experience, knowledge, attitudes and behaviour among different groups of males, rather than quantitative research, is what is missing to better understand male health issues. In the absence of a national move to seek evidence-based ways of promoting male health effectively, a research function to evaluate local pilot projects is essential, especially in health authority areas with no university within their boundaries.

International agencies

World Health Organization

The WHO's European Health For All (HFA) programme recently published its revised strategy, 'Health21: the Health For All Policy for the WHO European Region', which includes new targets for the 21st century. Although equity is one of the guiding principles of the HFA movement, women's issues have historically dominated the gender agenda within it, whilst males have never been recognised as a priority population group in relation to inequalities in health within the WHO European region.

European HFA targets for the 21st century were put out to consultation between September 1997 and March 1998. Several responses called for a clearer perspective on gender as the focus had previously been too women-centred and too biological in emphasis. They also suggested that a gender perspective in public health and health policy implied more than the prevention of ill health among males and females and should include the question of their respective roles in society.

An early draft of the revised targets had specified one on sex differences in health. However, this was removed following consultation responses from state members of the European HFA Network, some of whom commented that it overemphasised women's health. Others consulted proposed a clear linkage between the target on sex difference and other targets, such as those on population groups, violence and accidents, mental health and risky health behaviours, in order to take account of the different health experiences and outcomes for males and females in each case. One member state suggested the incorporation of a gender perspective in all relevant targets instead of the proposed sex inequality target.

The number of targets has been reduced from 38 to 21 and there are three that relate to specific population groups: babies and children, young people and the over 65s. From the perspective of sex and gender, the result of the consultation was that 'gender-sensitivity' apparently runs through the revised strategy and targets as a key value. This is defined as the:

> incorporation of a gender perspective into health policies and strategies. A gender perspective leads to a better understanding of the facts that influence the health of women and of men. It is not only concerned with biological differences between women and men, or with women's reproductive role, but acknowledges the effects of the socially, culturally and behaviourally determined relationships, roles and responsibilities of men and women, especially on individual, family and community health. (WHO, 1998b, p. 211)

However, it is not always apparent that this key value of gender-sensitivity – that encouragingly echoes how this publication defines sex-specificity and gender-sensitivity – has been integrated into all relevant targets regarding male health needs.

The major reference to sex inequalities in health is in the introduction to the new HFA policy, where the report discusses Target 2 Equity in Health among groups within countries, and states:

> There are great differences in health between men and women in the Region. . . . All sectors of society should assume responsibility for the reduction of social and gender inequities, and the alleviation of their consequences on health. (WHO, 1998a)

Target 2, Equity in Health, stipulates that:

> By . . . 2020, the health gap between socio-economic groups within countries should be reduced by at least one fourth in all member states, by sub-

stantially improving the level of health of disadvantaged groups. (WHO, 1998b)

The full policy report continues that: 'This target can be achieved if … public policies are … gender-sensitive.' (WHO, 1998b)

Out of the 21 targets, Target 2 is the only one with a specific reference to the health needs of males at the population level (WHO, 1998a). Significantly, reference to males is omitted from the following targets.

- Target 3 – *Healthy Start in Life*: where, for example, parents and mothers are mentioned, but not fathers.
- Target 4 – *Health of Young People* and Target 12 – *Reducing Harm from Alcohol, Drugs and Tobacco*: in relation to the numbers of lung cancer deaths among males and to male consumption of alcohol and drugs.
- Target 5 – *Healthy Ageing*: in relation to male life expectancy and disability-free life expectancy.
- Target 6 – *Improving Mental Health*: in relation to suicide among men.
- Target 7 – *Reducing Communicable Diseases*: in relation to HIV infection and AIDS among gay and bisexual men.
- Target 8 – *Reducing Noncommunicable Diseases*: in relation to male deaths from heart disease, stroke and cancer, especially of the lung and stomach.
- Target 9 – *Reducing Injury from Violence and Accidents*: in relation to male deaths due to accidents, e.g. at work, and violence, in particular homicide, and in relation to males as perpetrators of both, e.g. road traffic accidents and domestic violence.
- Target 13 – *Settings for Health*: in relation to male-dominated workplaces and, for example, accidents. (European Commission, 1995; WHO, 1998b)

Targets 2 and 3 are the only two targets that name women, but not men. Target 3, Healthy Start in Life, Target 4, Health of Young People and Target 5, Healthy Ageing are the population group-specific targets for the 21st century. Only Target 3 actually mentions one sex as a population group. Not surprisingly, it specifically refers to women's health and mothers in relation to policies and programmes concerning reproductive health care and child health services. It does refer to the importance of a supportive family and of parenting abilities and to community action in relation to abused children, although neither working with fathers and fathering nor with male perpetrators, respectively, is mentioned (WHO, 1998b).

Target 9, Reducing Injury from Violence and Accidents, is the only other target with a reference to so-called gender-sensitivity in its list of objectives. Whilst it does not name men or women, the target seeks reductions in mortality and disability in relation to seven categories of violence and accidents that affect males and females differently. Depending on how some of these terms are defined, males, for example, are predominantly affected by four of these: road traffic, work and leisure accidents and organised violence. Females are predominantly affected by three: domestic accidents, domestic and gender-related violence (European Commission, 1995; WHO, 1998b).

Various statistical indicators are listed in order to be able to measure performance towards meeting each target. Sex-specificity, or disaggregation by sex, is given as a requirement when collecting and analysing data for 8 out of the 21 targets, including for those relating to population groups. Yet, 'reported cases of gender, i.e. sex, related violence' is the only sex-specific indicator listed for monitoring progress with Target 9. This may possibly be because sex-specific data are not available for cases of violence and accidents, but this seems unlikely. Disaggregation by sex is not required for the remaining Targets, 12 and 13 out of a total of 11 that affect European Union males and females differently. Part of the explanation for this could be that the WHO European HFA Region takes in more countries now than the EU did in 1994, when there were 12 member states, all in Western Europe (WHO, 1998b).

The European Commission

An investigation during 1994/95 of the European Commission's public health policy revealed that neither sex figured as a population group receiving priority: the health of men was not, for example, on the agenda for the 1995 or 1996 work programme. Moreover, it was unclear how the European Commission (EC) viewed sex differences in health in comparison with variations across other influencing factors, e.g. age, social deprivation etc. The EC tended up until then to select topics (for health status reports) rather than target groups within the population. According to Commission officials (Williamson, 1997a), the selection of one population group and not another did not imply a lack of recognition of the latter's particular needs.

This appeared to be contradicted by other EC documentation, in which priority population groups were identified by age and social deprivation. Secondly, EU target groups had usually been identified as migrants, women, prisoners, young people and other socially deprived groups.

This did not apparently mean at the time that the EC was failing to recognise male health needs at the population level, as they were being addressed by programmes aimed at preventing the major public health scourges across the whole population. This included diseases and conditions of particular relevance for men and women. However, it was also unclear whether men and women were approached differently or in the same way within such programmes.

The Swiss Men's Health Charter

Outside the European Union, but still within Europe, strategic activity has been taking place in Switzerland with the creation of the Swiss Men's Health Charter. This task is being carried out by a small network of about seven professionals interested in male health issues facilitated by Dr Ulrich J. Grueninger of the Swiss Federal Office of Public Health (equivalent to the Health Ministry). The group has undertaken this work voluntarily in a deliberate effort to make it a healthy and sustainable process whilst being aware that such change requires much time.

The charter was successfully launched at a regional one day seminar on 30 April 1998. The seminar was introduced and closed by the Health Minister for the Canton (State) of Berne and a prominent (woman) Member of Parliament in Switzerland, respectively. Presentations were also made by the Head of Health Statistics at the Swiss Federal Office of Statistics, scientists from the Department of Preventive Medicine at the University of Zurich, the Swiss Foundation for Health Promotion, local health authorities, equal opportunity agencies, men's groups and other activists. Women guest speakers commented on the presentations.

The next step is to have the Swiss Health Foundation produce the final version, translate it into French and probably Italian and then distribute it widely across Switzerland. The network also applied for a grant from the Swiss Health Promotion Foundation to help fund this work.

Towards the end of 1998, the Health Strategy Development Unit took on a new responsibility: drafting a National Health Policy in Switzerland. It is expected that there will be opportunities to raise gender-specific health concerns during its development in 1999.

National and state men's health policies in Australia

Whilst the political system, government structures and policy-making processes may differ between Australia and the United Kingdom, both are western industrialised democracies and the broad picture of male health needs is very similar. There is also the similarity of sporadic and uncoordinated male health initiatives springing up across both countries within a national policy vacuum. Under the government of John Major, the Department of Health was made aware of the Australian draft national policy in 1996, but no official response was ever made.

Bearing these comparisons in mind along with the contemporary constitutional change in the UK that is expected to lead to regional government within England, it is informative to look more closely at the Australian experience and, in particular, at what the draft policy actually says. Lobbying Her Majesty's Government for a national male health policy may be neither appropriate nor realistic, but influencing it to ensure male health issues are named up front and integrated into all relevant national and regional health policies and policy-making processes is essential. Furthermore, by engaging men themselves in the consultation processes, Australian policy development at national and state level has encouraged greater ownership of the issues amongst males in the community. Achieving a similar awakening and connection in England would go a long way to securing effective public involvement in this major public health challenge.

The federal government

In the early 1990s, the Australian Labour federal government, under Bob Hawke, acknowledged a gap in national health policy on recognising that:

> Men's health, as a specific issue, has been gaining more attention in both the community and the health care field. Many of the major medical issues on the men's health agenda have long been receiving attention, and significant gains have been made.... [that] There has ... been activity in men's health initiatives by State Governments and at the community level, particularly by grassroots men's groups.... [but that] these achievements have not occurred as part of a co-ordinated national strategy within a clearly defined policy framework. (PHCG, 1996, p. 9)

The Federal Minister for Human Services and Health, Dr Carmen Lawrence, therefore instructed her department to organise the first national men's health conference in Australia. At the event, in August 1995, she announced the beginning of the development of a draft national men's health policy that:

> recommends a concerted approach by Federal, State and Territory Governments and community groups to tackle the high levels of preventable deaths, injuries, and illnesses experienced by various groups of Australian men. (Furler, 1996)

Initial consultation on the proposed policy initiative took place at this conference attended by over 500 delegates representing all states and territories; the health professions; all levels of government; community education and health services; service user and patient groups; and specific population groups, such as Aboriginal and Torres Strait Islander men, gay and bisexual men and men from non-English speaking backgrounds. Delegates commented on areas of priority for the policy to address and these included:

> the negative impacts of some aspects of male socialisation on risk-taking behaviour and in creating an unwillingness for men to talk about health or seek help ... the need for broad education strategies on the full range of men's

> health issues, involving schools, the media and workplaces; and ... the need
> to better target existing services to improve outcomes for men. (PHCG, 1996,
> pp. 10–11)

Further consultation on ideas for the national policy were tested in
November 1995 at a series of small forums held in Perth, Hobart, Adelaide,
Brisbane and Sydney – the capital cities of the main Australian states (only
excluding Canberra, ACT, where the federal government is based). These ·
forums reinforced the feedback from the national conference and the draft
policy was launched in January 1996. It advocated:

> an approach ... which acknowledges the wide range of influences on men's
> health, such as social, economic, psychological, cultural and biological fac-
> tors. For example, issues, such as the impact of masculinity and male
> socialisation on excessive risk-taking behaviour in young men and the impact
> of structural factors such as the nature of men's work, socio-economic status
> and unemployment, need to be considered. (Furler, 1996)

However, the plan to engage in formal, comprehensive consultation in early
1996 and complete the policy process by the end of that year was disrupted
by federal elections, in which Bob Hawke's Labour Party was heavily
defeated. Since then, and despite lobbying by many state governments and
individual and organisational male health advocates, the new Liberal
federal government has not seen fit to continue the policy development
process. The draft policy was, therefore, confined to the shelf to collect dust.

The draft policy includes sections on policy principles, national policy
context, goals, objectives, strategies in general and for boys and young men,
working age men and older men, performance indicators, roles and
responsibilities and an action plan that covers education, information and
research. Plans for monitoring, review and evaluation had not been
developed and further consultation was planned.

It is worth considering the applicability and transferability of certain
features of the policy to the situation in England, for example:

- the assumption that the health care system has always responded to the
  health needs of boys and men, who have few, if any, significant needs;
- the emergence of evidence that many male health needs, especially of
  those of particular groups of men, have been overlooked;
- the successful gendering of health care and policy from the female
  perspective that serves to illuminate the lack of critical examination
  from male perspectives;
- the need, firstly, to understand sex differences in mortality, morbidity
  and use of health services and what causes them within a social model of
  health and illness and, secondly, to adopt a primary health care
  approach in order to promote better male health and more responsive
  health services.

A social view of health recognises that social, economic, cultural and political factors, which lie outside the health system, make a major contribution to patterns of health and illness among population groups, including men. Effective prevention strategies must, therefore, involve partnerships with sectors outside health and have a long-term focus on change (PHCG, 1996, p. 39).

A primary health care approach recognises that the issues and health problems experienced by men are best tackled by services, which are located close to where men live and work and which integrate the provision of personal care and treatment with local public health and health promotion activities. Effective primary health care is built on the effective involvement of men and the wider community in the identification of needs, the development of strategies to meet those needs, and the ongoing management, monitoring and evaluation of those strategies and services (PHCG, 1996, p. 39).

In this context, primary health care is defined more broadly than the English status quo of primary health services provided by GPs and their practice colleagues, on the one hand, and of community health services by community nurses and other allied health professions, on the other. Such an approach envisages greater co-ordination of such services in partnership with other health-related community services (perhaps, even under one roof), more community involvement and a shift in emphasis from traditional core medical services to preventive services and a public health approach in primary care. There is food for thought here in relation to Healthy Living Centres, a proposal underpinned by the principles behind, and lessons learned by, the Peckham Health Centre model (Pearse and Crocker, 1943).

Whilst the Liberal federal government has so far been reluctant to pursue the idea of a national men's health policy, it is funding three national developments: a national men's health research agenda, a database on men's health initiatives, and a national centre for excellence in men's sexual and reproductive health. In addition, the Commonwealth House of Representatives Standing Committee on Family and Community Affairs held a seminar on male health issues in September 1997 (HRSCFCA, 1997).

South Australia

Although South Australia was the first state to begin developing a state-wide policy, it was, unfortunately, not the first state to launch and begin implementing its policy at the time of researching this section of this book. As with the national situation, politics intervened, this time in the form of state elections. What is of particular interest in this case study is the approach taken in the policy development process and, in particular, during the consultation phases.

One month after the first national men's health conference in 1995, the South Australian Health Commission officially sanctioned the proposed development of a state-wide men's health policy. This was in recognition that:

the health needs of men as a population group have not been given specific attention and not been addressed in a coherent and unified policy. This has allowed the health outcomes for men and the experiences and perceptions that men have of their health to remain largely unexamined. . . . [and] that men represent a diverse group with diverse health needs who also share some common patterns of health and illness. (SPPB, 1997, p. 4)

Initially, a steering committee was formed. Its terms of reference were: to steer forward the development of a draft policy and strategic directions paper for the state health system; to co-ordinate a consultation process on the draft paper; and to integrate the addressing of male health needs into the official service planning and development procedures of the entire state health system.

The steering committee then convened nine reference groups on a range of male health issues. In 1996, these groups produced papers on the following issues: the health of young males; the health of males from non-English speaking backgrounds; the health of rural males; males, accidents and injuries; males and violence; the health of gay males and homosexually active males; the health of older males; males and mental health; and males and suicide. These papers were produced to help identify the main issues in male health and to inform the development of the male health background paper that was to launch the official consultation process.

A particular challenge to the South Australia Health Commission was how to address the health needs of rural males. In this state, many males live in small or isolated communities, where geographical isolation is compounded by the limited availability or accessibility of various services. As Bentley and Booth (1995) wrote: 'One of the best ways of finding out how we can assist men is to ask them' (p. 37).

In the state's rural areas, therefore, the Commission's Country Health Services Division went on to hold male health forums, the aim of which was to:

provide a venue for men to have a say about what issues affect them and how the health system could help them prevent illness and maintain good health. (Bentley and Booth, 1995, p. 38)

At these events, male health issues were identified through words and music, guest speakers presented information on specific topics and facilitators encouraged further discussion in small groups. Issues included the role of males; how males are socialised; rural isolation; anger and violence; lifestyle factors; the nature of health services for males; and providing positive role models for young males in their relationships with others.

In mid 1997, the South Australian Health Commission published its first male health consultation paper. Later that year, state elections stopped the policy development in its tracks. At a meeting following the elections, the possibility of forming a new, broader committee on male health and family life to reflect the replacement of a state Minister for Health with one for Health, Housing and Family Services was proposed. However, this would then have meant a further delay of at least 18 months to put a new policy framework in place.

Wherever the policy process goes from then, the steering committee made considerable progress through an enlightened and refreshing approach to a newly recognised, yet little understood, complex and potentially controversial issue.

In order to ensure the final policy was as responsive, inclusive and equitable as it could be, the policy development framework was based on certain key principles:

- a social view of health;
- acknowledgement of the 'social construction of masculinities' and of the context of female health;
- equity;
- co-operative and co-ordinated action;
- community participation;
- reorienting health services;
- health promotion, information and education.

An understanding of masculinities in order to inform how best to address male health needs was fundamental to developing policy in this area from a social health perspective. Yet, the relationship between masculinities and the health status of males is seldom a feature of policy and practice to promote the health of boys and men in England. A 'social construction of masculinities' supports the following perspectives:

> ... there are diverse expressions of masculinity not a singular one ... men interpret their experiences of masculinity in relation to their race, ethnicity, socio-economic status, age, ability, sexuality and geographical location ... these interpretations and the values they express are not fixed and change over time ... some forms of masculinity are more dominant ... [and] ... the values of the masculinities are evident in men's health behaviour, their social and cultural practices and in the social structure. (SPPB, 1997, p. 7)

The implications of adopting these principles for policy development were the need to:

> understand how men, who accept the dominant idea of masculinity, perceive and respond to illness, and how they adopt health related practices and use the health system ... [and] how men, who have differing interpretations of masculinity, are affected by the dominant expression and similarly how these groups perceive health, respond to illness and how they adopt health related practices and use the health system. (SPPB, 1997, p. 12)

Another aspect of the work in South Australia that might be usefully adapted in the UK is the policy development experience being, for those males playing a part in it:

> part of the process of men critically examining their male identities and ... an expression of a social process of men involved in redefining their identities. (SPPB, 1997, p. 12)

For example, a deliberate attempt was made, when setting the steering group up, to conduct proceedings with a heightened sense of awareness of the influence of the dominant form of masculinity upon its work within an institution, where positions of power tend to be male-dominated. This not only meant ensuring women were also members of the committee and that female health services and the women's movement were represented, but also that male members engaged both professionally and personally in the committee's discussions.

The South Australian Health Commission paper is quite clear in its views.

> If we are to gain a more complete picture of the ways that men respond to illness, we also need to know what meanings they construct about terms such as health. Ethnic and racial variations are obvious examples, where differences can be found. Young men also have different health priorities to older men ... ... however, the research evidence that could help inform a men's health policy is not easily found. (SPPB, 1997, p. 53)

It concludes by raising important questions for the future such as that expressed above, that are relevant to the situation in England. An effective policy, it continues:

> must have a range of strategies to meet the differing interpretations, circumstances and health needs of men ... [and] must be able to understand and work from within men's interpretations as far as possible. (SPPB, 1997, p. 12)

New South Wales

The 1995 state elections in New South Wales (NSW) elected a Labour government. Not long after the first national men's health conference that same year, the new state administration committed itself to working, on the one hand, with the Labour federal government on male health policy and, on the other, with local groups to develop a response at state level. However, developments within NSW were delayed following the change to a Liberal federal government at the national level. This had led to no further action being taken with the draft national men's health policy published under the previous Labour government in early 1996.

As was the case nationally, male health became a higher profile issue in NSW amongst both health and other service providers and the wider community, including the local media. Many local male health activities had sprung up. The need for a state men's health strategy was apparent as:

> a common message [had] arisen: workers and agencies are looking for a guiding framework for their work with men. (MHPAC, 1998, Foreword)

So, in early 1997, the NSW Health Department set up a Men's Health Policy Advisory Committee at ministerial level. The committee membership comprised academics, key public servants, ministerial advisers, a Labour Party MP and a feminist academic. It steered the preparation of a discussion paper, which represented: 'a first step in developing a consistent and prioritised approach to addressing men's health issues in NSW' (Reid, 1998).

In order to prepare the discussion paper, all health services and related governmental and non-governmental organisations in the state were surveyed to identify current health activity targeting males (MHPAC, 1998, p. 2).

The next steps in the policy development process included:

1. Consult other key informants.
2. Internal seminars for interested officers within the Department of Health in order to build wider ownership of the policy. This resulted in a clearer focus to the development process and generated anticipation within the department.
3. Draft discussion paper submitted to the Department's Policy Development Committee. The committee's official endorsement of the paper ensured the support of senior departmental staff.
4. Meetings with representatives from other departments, for whose work some of the recommendations had implications. This helped break down barriers as well as build wider ownership.
5. Ministerial approval and an official media launch by the Minister for Health. The mainstream press covered it and some men's magazines expressed interest in becoming involved with recommended work.
6. Wider consultation included: publishing the discussion paper; circulating it throughout the health system, i.e. the 17 statutory Area Health Services, other departments, other states, academia, male health organisations, GPs and specialist men's clinics; making it available on

websites, e.g. of the Department of Health and of a number of men's organisations; and, seeking community feedback in writing and through being invited to local meetings.

7. Area Health Services to take the discussion paper through their standard planning and consultation processes in preparation for the modification of local service delivery within the parameters of the overarching state policy.
8. Analysis of responses to the discussion paper: many enthusiastic and positive comments were received in response to a request for information and ideas.
9. Revision of the discussion paper to produce a final official strategy in light of this and other feedback.
10. Launch of the New South Wales State Men's Health Strategy: planned for 1999.

At the time of researching this case study, all the recommended strategies in the discussion paper had been officially approved for implementation. Moreover, funding had been allocated for a variety of research projects. It was also intended that a Men's Health Information and Referral Centre be set up with state funding. The function of the centre would be to promote male health and to advise the Department on male health. Further limited, but recurrent, funding was also expected to be allocated for new initiatives, staff education and training and ongoing research.

The strategic approach preferred by the NSW Department of Health is one of reorienting the delivery of health care services and the systems supporting these services rather than prioritising specific diseases. This is reflected in the strategy's central tenets that are to recognise that:

> some groups of men require more assistance and support than others. . . . By improving the health and health behaviours of men, the health of other members of the community will also benefit. (MHPAC, 1998, p. 1)

These tenets also include enabling male participation in service planning, on the one hand, and health professionals to consider gender issues from male perspectives when designing and delivery services on the other, as well as promoting partnerships between the health care sector and non-health sectors, including the voluntary sector, to stimulate innovatory practice to better the health of males in greatest need and promoting good practice once established. There is also a requirement for all organisations in the health community to identify and address male health needs; and supporting research is to be conducted into the relationship between gender, health behaviour, health outcomes and the development of health services (MHPAC, 1998, pp. 1–2).

The discussion paper also lays down principles to guide the development and implementation of the state strategy. These cover:

- adopting a holistic view of health and an evidence-based approach;
- building partnerships within the health sector and with non-health sectors;
- involving the community;
- targeting those in greater need and taking the diversity of needs within the male population into account, whilst also ensuring that other population groups, such as women and children, are not excluded;
- enabling health services to be more appropriate and accessible to males.

An additional element of the strategy development and implementation processes, that relates to the principle of community involvement, is the specific involvement of males. The discussion paper:

> is the first stage in seeking men's input. As the ... men's health strategy progresses, agencies must find appropriate ways to engage men in planning and delivering services that meet their needs. (MHPAC, 1998, p. 7)

Engaging and involving males has been a key feature in the development of both policy and practice in Australia. It is fundamental to their appropriateness and effectiveness and represents a highly relevant transferable principle to the situation in the UK. It would also go some way to interesting greater numbers of males in their own health. To date, however, whereas many of the relatively small number of male health initiatives have consulted local boys or men during their planning stages, there are few examples of policy development work that have specifically targeted males across the population.

Conclusion

Men's health has evolved into a far higher profile issue in Australia than in England within the health sector, the political sphere and the broader public arena. Grassroots activity, academic research and advocacy work regarding a range of issues to do with boys and men and masculinities have mushroomed in Australia in the 1990s with their roots going back into the 1970s. From the strategic perspective, it is worthwhile taking a closer look at men's health policy in Australia to consider the transferability of any principles, practice and lessons learned to England. However, Lumb (1998) is not optimistic in his critique of men's health policy in his country.

> It should be noted that to date [late 1997] there has been no men's health policy implementation in Australia and it is my assessment that, despite some policy formulation work, the current prognosis for men's health programs is dim. (Lumb, 1998)

The federal government of Australia held the first national men's health conference in Melbourne in August 1995. At the event, Dr Carmen

Lawrence, Federal Minister for Human Services and Health, launched the initiative for a national men's health policy. A second national conference was held in Perth in October/November 1997 and a third is being planned for the year 2000 in the Northern Territories. Men's health policy development and programme activity in several states and territories were stimulated by this major conference. One state, South Australia, had already got its policy development process under way. Unfortunately, both the national and the South Australian attempts to develop men's health policy fell foul of the bigger political picture.

Other states have since taken up the challenge, notably New South Wales, Western Australia and Tasmania. Case studies were presented in this book on South Australia and on New South Wales, as the policy experience to date had been fuller in those states.

The Health Department of Western Australia published its State Men's Health Policy in 1997. Its aim is to:

provide an overarching framework for future action aimed at men's health for different levels of government, as well as non-government, professional and education/research agencies. (HDWA, 1997, p. 25)

Although the process involved to develop this policy did not involve extensive, state-wide consultation in the same way as occurred in other states, the policy was: 'prepared with the help of a number of key clinical consumer and community stakeholders with an interest in men's health' (HDWA, 1997, p. 3).

Progress in Tasmania is still more recent. In 1998, the Tasmanian Department of Community and Health Services appointed a Policy Officer. The initial task for this post was to collect and analyse epidemiological data and conduct a literature search. The policy development process would be integral to the overall work of the department, so that, for example, departmental protocols on community consultation are applied when conducting consultations regarding men's health. Key principles of the policy development process include: establishing an advisory group at the highest possible level, i.e. reporting to the state minister, that comprises a cross section of the community; encouraging positive media coverage; and conducting extensive and sophisticated consultation.

Having explored national and state-level experience of developing male health policy in Australia, we emphasise ten key transferable issues for consideration when planning policy and strategy at local level in England, e.g. at health authority level in relation to Health Improvement Programmes:

- the justification and rationale for a coherent and unified policy for the male population;
- the potential contribution of the overarching function of a male health

policy umbrella to the development of appropriate and effective responses to male health needs at the local level;

- the need for, and benefits of, comprehensive and extensive consultation with all interested agencies at all levels and especially with boys and men in the community;
- the principle of inclusiveness as a response to the diversity of boys, young men and older men and, therefore, of their health-related needs – and the consequent implication of how best to reach and engage groups of males, traditionally defined as 'hard to reach', in a consultation process;
- the link between consulting boys and men and each individual male's engagement with the issues;
- an approach that recognises the breadth of influences on the health status of males;
- the relevance of an understanding of masculinities and their relationship to health-related attitudes, behaviour and experience;
- the principles of integrating directions in male health policy into all other relevant health strategy and project activity;
- the urgent need to draw up a national male health research agenda with an emphasis on qualitative research into boys' and men's experiences of health and wellbeing;
- a focus on reorienting health service systems and structures rather than on prioritising disease topics.

In the Australian context, promising policy development processes have occurred – albeit at the more highly politicised levels of national and state government than at the local level of a health authority in England that we are advocating. They have also revealed common principles for those interested in men's health policy to reflect upon. Unfortunately, evidence of successful implementation of such policies is so far lacking. Furthermore, according to Lumb (1997):

> men's health policy activity is not ... a part of any internationally sustained political activity, and nor is there an emerging critique of contemporary health practice from masculine perspectives, such that health institutions would be challenged to continue to change. (Lumb, 1998)

Lumb's critique of men's health policy in Australia draws on his experience of chairing the South Australian Men's Health Policy Steering Committee. His view is that progress with such policy is blocked by:

- the absence, and problematic nature, of a men's social movement;
- the current oversimplified popular discourse on male health issues, partly sustained by the media's competitive view of men's and women's health needs;
- on the one hand, the overreliance on quantitative, evidence-based data

on male health needs, and, on the other, the paucity of qualitative research into boys and men and their health;
- the influence of dominant masculine values (hegemonic masculinity) within policy making and other significant power structures and relations in society.

If there is room for optimism, Lumb concludes, men's health policies may see the light of day in the future, if:

> people on the margins, and people in the least secure social positions, in terms of education, occupational prestige, income and Aboriginality can get together, and get politically active. (Lumb, 1998)

Summary

The health needs of the male population in England are a major public health problem. Earlier chapters illustrate the breadth and depth of their nature and track their causes and roots back into the very fabric of our society and its history. Yet, as the new millennium dawns, only patchy progress has been made to tackle the problem. What is missing is a clear sense of what direction efforts to address these issues should go in.

We put forward the case for strategic development to fill the void, in which activities presently take place. 'Gendered' public health policy and programmes are required. The male dimension must be integrated into all relevant public health activity to take account not just of the biological factors relating to sex differences, but also of the implied psychological, social and cultural issues concerning living as a boy or man in today's society.

The NHS has traditionally provided preventive health services that have addressed the specific health needs of boys and men only in implicit and indirect ways with few notable exceptions, e.g. sexual health programmes among gay and bisexual men and, more recently, sex education classes for boys in schools. National developments in response to the official recognition of male health needs at the population level given by the then Chief Medical Officer (DOH, 1993) have been few and far between, although there has been some significant, small-scale government activity, e.g. at the Department of Health.

More recently, the emergence of national health policy during the 1990s has provided several opportunities to raise the profile of male health issues. However, it remains unclear where these sit – from the Labour government's point of view – within the narrow context of sex differences in health and the broader one of inequalities in health across society. Fortunately, the latest official investigation into health inequalities, the Independent Inquiry into Inequalities in Health, has made a valuable contribution towards the naming of male health needs as a public health problem (Acheson, 1998).

A more comprehensive and fully rounded picture has still to be painted: one that views boys and men more holistically, taking into account the major socio-economic changes affecting males in England today. Part of this picture will, it is hoped, be filled in by research studies such as those underway in the government funded Health Variations Programme.

What more is being and can be done? Whilst there seems little point in lobbying government for a national male health strategy – even though it may sometimes feel like a concrete and tangible aim – the New Labour government may prove more amenable to demands for such a strategy. By placing health inequalities centre-stage, government health policy should take gender (i.e. sex) inequalities in health, more seriously than the previous Conservative administrations. There is also evidence that broader social issues to do with boys and men and masculinities, e.g. educational underachievement, unemployment, crime and social exclusion, are becoming a more central political concern.

Within the health arena, *The New NHS* and *Our Healthier Nation* White Papers open up a variety of opportunities for the gendering of health policy and programmes from male perspectives. The submission and consultation processes for the Independent Inquiry into Inequalities in Health and the *Our Healthier Nation* Green Papers, respectively, were a first tentative step. Future opportunities for national and local leverage are highlighted.

Finally, it is informative to reflect upon experience in Europe and further afield in Australia, where national and state men's health policy has been developed, to consider what lessons can be learned and what may be transferable to England.

To what extent do you think Lumb's analysis (p. 181) resonates with the contemporary situation of male health strategy development in England?

The next chapter takes a more detailed look at the local level. It describes a variety of experiences – in England and Europe – as case studies and draws out common and different themes. With these local perspectives, and the national and international perspectives given in this chapter, in mind, Chapter 9 then develops some concrete ways forward for a strategic approach to addressing male health needs.

Further reading

Acheson, D. (1998) *Independent Inquiry into Inequalities in Health.* The Stationery Office, London.

DOH (1998) *Chief Medical Officer's Project to Strengthen the Public Health Function in England – Report of emerging findings.* The Stationery Office, London.

NHSE (1995) *Variations in Health: Report of the Variations Sub-Group of the Chief Medical Officer's Health of the Nation Working Group.* National Health Service Executive, Leeds.

Chapter 8
Local Perspectives

In this chapter we:

- introduce and outline strategic development activity at the levels of the regional office and the health authority within the NHS;
- describe, in more detail, one regional health authority's attempt to address strategically the health needs of boys and men within its population;
- describe case studies of health authorities and case studies of efforts initiated by agencies outside the NHS, e.g. local men's health networks;
- describe four European case studies;
- reflect on the factors that, on the one hand, supported local attempts to get male health needs addressed and, on the other, became obstacles.

Introduction

This chapter brings the focus down from the national to the local level. It will examine the work of a variety of organisations and agencies and consider the results of their advocacy for a more direct and effective response by the NHS (in particular, by health authorities) to address the health needs of local men. One regional health authority (now a regional office of the NHS Executive), over ten (former district) health authorities and six non-NHS bodies are reported on as specific case studies, where substantial activity was initiated and useful insight can be gleaned. The actual documentation of these case studies is a significant step in itself, as much of the male health work in England to date has not been reported on.

The West Midlands case study describes work stimulated by the Director of Public Health for the then West Midlands Regional Health Authority (now the NHS Executive – West Midlands) through his 1994 report. This was the first major public health report from within the NHS since the Chief Medical Officer's 'State of the Public Health' report for 1992 to cover male health as a major theme. It led to the only top-down initiative by an NHS region intended to encourage its health authorities to tackle male health needs at the population level more effectively. Its impact is illustrated mainly through responses to the initiative made by health authorities within the West Midlands.

Two further NHS case studies are then presented, this time from the East Midlands. In one, strategic development was sought within a health authority by attempting to move male health needs higher up the organisation's agenda in response to the national situation. In the other, strategic activity came about as a result of particular local health trends (that happened to affect males) being identified.

To complement NHS activity, case studies on agencies independent of the NHS are then described. Local men's health networks (numbering ten in England as of early 1999) continue to play a vital role in raising the profile of male health issues and seeking action to address them. Three are covered here, including the first to arrive on the scene, the East Midlands Men's Health Network. The efforts of a national body and a single issue charity are also briefly discussed.

Reflecting on the combined experience of these examples, two sections highlight factors supportive of, and factors causing obstacles to, strategic development in response to male health needs. Some factors may seem inevitable, whereas others may be amenable to intervention.

Finally, to bring an international perspective, short local case studies are given from Germany, Austria and the Republic of Ireland.

Below the national level

The impetus for action

As has already been suggested, the evolution of male health as a social issue has different origins and male health is not taking the same path as female health did. It cannot be characterised as either a top-down or bottom-up development. There has been no distinguishable men's movement pushing the issues up the popular and political agenda as was the case with the women's movement and female health issues.

The impetus for action to be taken on male health issues appears to have built up through a growing and relatively recent realisation amongst various 'observers' and 'witnesses'. Observers have included people in a position to be able to look at the big picture of health trends across whole populations, such as public health professionals, e.g. epidemiologists. Witnesses have included grassroots workers in different fields: health, education, probation and social services in the public sector along with independent practitioners and volunteers involved in self-help and, broadly speaking, caring agencies in the private sector. Many observers and witnesses came together with the formation of local men's health networks or forums from the late 1980s onwards. Others, especially witnesses, continued to work away in relative isolation and with little support from above, e.g. from direct line management.

There is little evidence of lay engagement, although a few small-scale examples do exist. Kirklees Men's Health Network was established under the auspices of the local Health For All network and programme, where community involvement was encouraged from the beginning. Another example is one of the conferences held in the 1990s that stands out as an exception in involving the community: the Gender and Health Conference (Glasgow Healthy City Project, 1994) where there was equal participation by lay and professional people. Unfortunately this did not lead to further action regarding the health of local men, although at least two male health projects were started in the local communities in the early to mid 1990s. A final example of public involvement, this time from overseas, can be found in the recent consultative work carried out by the North Western Health Board in the Republic of Ireland, described later in this chapter.

There are also a small number of self-help charities, e.g. the Men's Health Trust, that have been set up to respond to the health needs of men, but these have usually been single issue organisations predominantly focusing on different aspects of male-specific sexual health, e.g. prostate cancer, incontinence and impotence.

Momentum has gradually been gathering since the mid to late 1980s, but more rapidly since circa 1993, as awareness of male health issues has become more widespread throughout society. Women have spoken from their own experience of the worsening health of the men and boys in their lives to bring attention to the issues. Some men have become involved in personal and social development activity as a result of their recognising the need to try to change their own situation. The publishing industry has responded to part of the growing popular interest – the part principally interested in improving body image and sexual performance – in male health issues by launching three new men's lifestyle magazines in 1995. A number of more comprehensive factual self-help books have also been published (see Chapter 1).

However, at the time of publication, there remains only limited, patchy and often confused professional and lay knowledge of male health issues. Moreover, no clear definition of male health has yet been found.

NHS activity at regional and district level

Within the NHS, strategic planning and policy development activity regarding the health needs of males as a population group has remained the exception rather than the rule both at the former regional and at health authority level. Some of the earliest official reporting of male health needs only occurred in the last decade. One example is the chapter on male health in *Our City, Our Health: Ideas for improving health in Sheffield*, a consultative document produced by Healthy Sheffield 2000 in 1991 (Halliday, 1991). Perhaps the first male health initiative to be implemented, 'Better Health for Men', began in Glasgow in the 1980s.

At the time of publication, the former West Midlands Regional Health Authority (RHA) was alone among other RHAs, now regional offices of the NHS Executive, in having highlighted male health as a major public health problem and in having taken steps to enable the health authorities (HAs) within its region to begin to address the issue. This is, perhaps, the only major top-down example of strategic activity to date within the NHS.

It commissioned consultancy services from the London-based agency Working With Men to help health authorities address male health from the sociological and the epidemiological perspectives. Three stages were involved in this planning work: a regional seminar for representatives from all health authorities; consultancy at health authority level to begin planning for male health; and, recommendations for further research and development and for monitoring the impact of plans.

A number of health authorities have responded to the CMO's recommendation in 1993 to find out how best to promote male health. Only a handful of public health and health promotion interventions designed specifically with men in mind are in evidence on the ground. The major exceptions are the widespread HIV prevention, treatment and care programmes among gay men, bisexual men and men who have sex with men, and also sex education programmes among boys in schools.

The first health authority public health report to devote a whole chapter to the health of men was that of the Director of Public Health for Calderdale and Kirklees in 1996 (Worth, 1997). It made six relevant recommendations, five of which were:

- to further investigate male health needs in order to set priorities for future provision of local health services;
- to ensure the delivery of health promotion schemes at appropriate and accessible locations;
- to advise GPs to include male health in their health promotion activities;
- to build links with other men's health networks in the UK and Europe;
- to support a conference organised by the Kirklees Men's Health Network to identify ways forward.

Local reaction to the issues raised in the chapter was significant and mostly affirmative. This included both interest in the health authority's general approach to sex differences in health from the Department of Health and, specifically, in Kirklees Men's Health Network activities from neighbouring Calderdale (Worth, 1998).

The first health authority public health report to have male health as its main theme was that of the Director of Public Health for Nottingham Health Authority in 1998 (Wilson, 1999) discussed later in the chapter.

Health authorities – West Midlands

A major regional NHS initiative

The Regional Director of Public Health highlighted male health needs and that something should be done to address them in his annual report for 1994. The West Midlands Regional Health Authority then commissioned the London-based agency, Working With Men, to provide consultancy both to the region and to the health authorities within it in order to take its recommendations forward.

This resulted, first, in a day-long regional men's health seminar held in December 1995 for health authority representatives. There was a mixed representation from authorities across the region, with some authorities not represented. Second, the majority of authorities then used the regional funded consultancy for similar events locally, or to commission literature reviews.

Work specific to male health issues is now taken forward by local health authorities with only one regional initiative in place, the 'Men who have sex with men' project, which is funded through a regional levy.

In order to try to identify strategic policy development at health authority level within the West Midlands following the consultancy input, attempts were made to contact all health authorities that sent representatives to the regional seminar in 1995. In situations where the representative was no longer in post, contact was made with a senior member of the authority's public health department or local health promotion service. In all, information was obtained from 9 out of the 13 Health Authorities in the NHSE–West Midlands area.

One step forward and two steps back

In Worcestershire Health Authority, the regionally funded consultancy was used to organise a local conference on male health for interested professionals in March 1996. A joint Worcestershire and Herefordshire Health Authority meeting for health promotion and public health staff was also held in order to produce a male health strategy for the two counties. Workshops then took place for health workers and teachers in January 1997 in response to their expressed needs for support regarding sex education among boys and young men and for health service delivery among males, respectively. No further progress was made with these initiatives.

A second attempt to address male health issues locally involved a conference in 1997 on young men in the educational setting, 'Are they being served: Young men's needs in a school context'. Jointly organised by the local education authority (LEA) and the health authority, it succeeded in identifying ways forward. However, no plans were subsequently implemented.

In the same year, a male mentor project, co-ordinated by Hereford and Worcester Age Concern Ageing Well, had been set up as a partnership between Age Concern district groups, Herefordshire and Worcestershire Health Authorities and local GPs. This project seeks to target men over 50 to promote their physical and mental health and wellbeing through peer group counsellors and senior health mentors.

Worcestershire Health Authority health promotion objectives for 1998/9 to improve the health of males include:

- auditing the activity of local programmes designed to meet Health Improvement Programme objectives relevant to males;
- reviewing educational initiatives aimed at promoting boys' and young men's achievement;
- setting up a local men's health network to raise awareness of the health, social and educational needs of males;
- assessing the health information needs of frontline service providers.

Further plans at the health authority level were reported as uncertain at the time of writing this chapter (Johnson, 1998).

Raising awareness

Solihull Health Authority used the regionally funded consultancy to pay for a workshop for public health professionals and health service purchasers and another for health service providers, both run jointly with Coventry Health Authority. It is unclear what impact this consultancy had. Whilst the local workshop was well received and the issues raised made a positive impression, it is difficult to identify any further, concrete developments. Male health issues were raised, however, in a section of the Director of Public Health's annual report for 1995/6 that concludes:

> The challenge is to understand men's needs, hopes and fears and to develop the right approaches and services for them through the imaginative use of [health service] commissioning processes. (Cooper, 1996)

Unfortunately, no further work was taken forward between 1996 and 1998. In primary care, for example, male health needs have tended to be responded to only on a reactive basis. Future plans are likely to include the authority's first Health Improvement Programme acting as a vehicle to promote good men's health practice. Subsequent versions of the pro-gramme over the coming years will focus on different health topics thus presenting further opportunities to move male health forward. Another section on male health is to be included in the Director of Public Health's annual report for 1998/9.

Independent local action

Coventry Health Authority used the regional moneys for joint workshops with Solihull Health Authority (see above). Whilst research for this section identified no further local action specifically leading on from these events, significant developments took place not long afterwards.

Some attention was paid to the health of young men in the form of funding new projects and posts. This occurred in response to local issues, but not within a population-based male health strategy. The high incidence of suicide was addressed through funding a theatre-in-education project and the employment of a consultant psychotherapist with a special interest in the area. In 1997, a specialist health promotion post with a remit for young men was also created. However, due to the existing lack of local health promotion support and infrastructure regarding the health needs of young people, in general, the postholder was required to take on wider responsibilities for young men and women.

Another initiative, the 'Alive and Kicking' project, was implemented in 1996/7 by Coventry Education Development Centre in partnership with Coventry and Leicester Health Authorities and Coventry City Football Club. The project was part-funded by a grant from the Department of Health and aimed:

> to improve young men's health by working with two Sunday football leagues to raise awareness about healthy lifestyles. (CEDC, 1997)

Whilst this pilot project started after the regional men's health seminar and was active at the time of the joint Coventry and Solihull Health Authority workshops, it was not related to the regional initiative.

Recommendations not implemented

Recommendations to invest in addressing male health needs at the popu-lation level, whilst initially agreed by North Staffordshire Health Authority, were not actually implemented. Sexual health programmes among gay and bisexual males remain the only major male-specific activities on the ground, but these did not evolve out of the regional male health initiative.

No further strategic policy developments have occurred here and no plans to do so were in place for the future at the time of researching this chapter.

Regional monies not used

It appears that the regional funding for the Herefordshire Health Authority to use the consultancy to take male health forward locally was not used.

Whilst the health authority recognises male health needs at the population level, the regional initiative did not lead to any specific strategic or policy development activity. Coronary heart disease, however, is a major public health problem in Herefordshire and preventive interventions do target males, albeit implicitly.

The Director of Public Health for Herefordshire stated that:

> [the] only area where we are particularly concentrating on men's health is our gay men's project.... As for other services, we tend not to consider whether the service is aimed at either men or women, although, depending on the service, obviously more men or more women use it. (Deakin, 1998)

Herefordshire Health Authority has, however, identified suicide as a local target to include in their first Health Improvement Programme. At the time of writing, it is not known whether this target will be sex-specific.

Sustained local advocacy

In the Warwickshire Health Authority area, at a meeting of the Health of the Nation group in October 1995, it was agreed that:

> consultation on the subject [men's health] would take place with a wide range of Health Authority and community based workers with the objective of producing a position paper. (Broad and Jenkins, 1996)

The regionally funded consultancy enabled a workshop to be held on 23 April 1996 for such consultation to take place. This workshop aimed to:

> identify what further work may need to be undertaken and consider any implications for purchasers and providers ... for consideration by the Health of the Nation Group. (Broad and Jenkins, 1996)

A report on the workshop was discussed at a further Health of the Nation group meeting that summer. The report included recommendations, such as that the group:

> acknowledge that there is a gender issue that requires addressing by the Health Authority and other agencies ... commission the development of a

strategic plan to tackle men's health issues … [and] ratify the Strategic Plan and make recommendations for further action. (Broad and Jenkins, 1996)

However, no steps were taken at the strategic level in response to these recommendations.

Another attempt to take things forward strategically was made in response to the autumn 1996 NHS conference on gender and health in London – a result of the government signing up to the UN commitment to mainstream gender into all policies and programmes. A second paper – this time focusing on broader gender and health issues – was discussed at a spring 1997 meeting of the Health of the Nation group. The paper called for and outlined:

a more in-depth approach to addressing gender sensitivity and gender specificity in purchasing and consequently service provision. (Broad and Jenkins, 1997)

This was intended to maximise the health authority's potential to reduce sex differences in the Health of the Nation key area targets. Once again, no strategic impact was apparent within the health authority. The paper was also presented at the South Warwickshire Community Health Council, but with little, if any, effect.

No further action

No further action was taken by South Staffordshire Health Authority following the regional seminar and there are no plans to do so in the future. Neither of the Sandwell Health Authority representatives at the regional seminar was still in post when this chapter was being researched. According to the Public Health Department and Health Promotion Unit, no further developments occurred. The Birmingham Health Authority representative, who attended the regional seminar, moved jobs in the interim. The regionally funded consultancy led to no further strategic work locally.

East Midlands

A dedicated men's health promotion programme

North Derbyshire Health Authority was perhaps the first in England to establish a specialist male health promotion programme area. This happened in 1995 as a result of programme area reorganisation and meant that a programme manager took this responsibility on as the main part of their remit. Up until this time, it had been more usual in the NHS for male health either not to be delegated to any health authority health promotion officer or specialist, or, more recently, for it to be tacked on to their job descriptions as a minor remit.

North Derbyshire Health Authority had already shown an initial commitment to addressing male health needs through its support of the East Midlands Men's Health Network (see below) and its activities. During the 1990s, those working in North Derbyshire became the majority of the network membership. In addition to this, the health promotion specialist, who was to take on the male health remit, had specialised in this sphere whilst studying for a Master of Public Health degree. This partly involved a study trip to Australia to investigate the transferability of principles and actual examples, of effective practice to England. Australia had, by that time, probably progressed further than any other industrialised country in its attempts to address male health issues.

The health authority's overall health promotion programme, initiated in the late 1980s, is based on a 'settings' approach within each of six geographical localities as well as across the whole district. There are four main settings: schools, colleges and youth service; workplace; NHS professionals; and the wider community. Priority population groups are then targeted through these programme areas. It has only been since the mid 1990s that topic- or population-based areas were introduced for mental health and men's health, respectively. Health promotion specialists work as programme managers or as locality health promotion co-ordinators.

Aspects of strategic development was the first piece of practice selected to be transferred from Australia into this health authority. In Australia, the track record, both nationally and at state level, since early 1994/5 in terms of drafting male health strategies has been impressive (see National and state men's health policies in Australia in Chapter 7). In North Derbyshire, an internal Health Promotion Service discussion paper was drafted and consulted on. However, the process faltered before a formal male health promotion policy could be produced and it did not immediately influence the authority's health promotion purchasing plan, the official strategic document.

Some developments did subsequently take place on the ground during 1995 and 1996, but not as a direct result of this attempt to influence strategy. The men's health programme area put a proposal together for a pilot project based on identified evidence of effectiveness. This led to the implementation of a men's waist reduction initiative as part of a randomised control trial of interventions to prevent heart disease. 'Waist Watchers' targeted 40- to 60-year-old men living in a former coalfields village of North Derbyshire. A similar scheme was then piloted in a local heavy industry. Waist Watchers was then developed further and extended out to other workplaces and community sites, such as working men's clubs and miners' welfare institutes.

The programme area has also been involved in supporting a Personal and Social Education Co-ordinator at a local comprehensive school. A day-long workshop, 'Boyswork', was held in June 1996 with 14/15-year-old boys to investigate ways of engaging them in discussions about contemporary issues relating to their health and identity (Williamson, 1997b).

The attempt to influence strategy was then widened in 1996 by the setting up of a time-limited small interdepartmental Gender and Health Working Group within the health authority, following the 1995 commitment by the UK government to a UN policy 'to mainstream gender into all policies and programmes'. The group met regularly to look at opportunities to highlight previously lacking male perspectives on gender and health issues in the health authority's activity. Two developments followed on from this work. First, the authority's 1996/7 research programme included qualitative, focus group research into different men's experience of health problems and of health services (Bond and Williamson, 1998). Recommendations from this research were approved by the health authority's executive directors in 1998 in order to take this work forward. They include a recommendation for further research into men and help-seeking behaviour in relation to the major public health problems affecting the local male population. Secondly, the authority's 1996 Public Health Report included a chapter on prostate cancer screening, diagnosis and treatment.

The Gender and Health Working Group had only a limited impact on health authority work. Meetings stopped in 1997. Efforts to integrate male perspectives into other health promotion programme areas and across localities in a systematic and meaningful way remain in their early days at the time of writing.

On a more positive note, this is one of the health authority areas where it has been possible to take things forward in a concrete and productive, but limited, way. The Health Authority's first Health Improvement Programme recognises gender, i.e. sex, as an important factor in relation to its target on local health inequalities. Further work is planned regarding this issue until mid 2001.

Local health report highlights male health

The health of the male population was selected as the main theme of the annual public health report for Nottingham Health District, because:

> it was clear from the information presented in the three previous reports, and following on from the emphasis given in the Chief Medical Officer's report on the state of the public health in 1992, that not enough importance has been given in Nottingham and in the United Kingdom overall to both analysing the health needs of men and addressing how any unmet health needs could be met. (Wilson, 1999, p. 2)

The report identifies heart disease and stroke among the local male population as:

> an area where we should concentrate our efforts on not only preventing the disease in the first place, but on reducing the impact of that disease. (Wilson, 1999, p. 2)

and acknowledges that:

> there is a problem with men taking opportunities for health promotion and disease prevention and ... giving the appropriate priority to adopting a healthier lifestyle. (Wilson, 1999, p. 2)

The significant and widening gap in heart disease deaths among local men is also highlighted. Following a chapter on the overall health status of the male population within the Nottingham Health District, the report covers employment, unemployment and health; risk-taking behaviour and health; sexual health; and mental health. It also discusses differences in the ways males and females use health services.

The report makes a total of 20 recommendations, just over half of which are gendered. A number of ways male health could be improved locally are identified, including:

- focusing on occupational asthma and contact dermatitis as major occupational health risks using a framework based on the 'healthy workplace' concept proposed in 'Our Healthier Nation';
- multi-agency partnership to deal with racial harassment;
- implementing initiatives to improve the accessibility and responsiveness of services to the health needs of unemployed people;
- research into the impact of risk taking among males on their health;
- the availability of appropriate health information in relevant settings;
- Primary Care Groups assessing the health needs of their local male population and commissioning services accordingly;
- health service providers reorienting the delivery of their services to local boys and men;
- better sex education in schools, at home, in youth clubs – and via outreach projects that can also provide advice and condoms to male teenagers – through a multi-agency approach;
- reviewing sexual dysfunction services for men;
- greater awareness of sex and gender when improving mental health services;
- developing programmes to enable men to manage their anger and aggressive behaviour more effectively;
- encouraging males to use preventive health services and ensuring these are available;

- ensuring equal access to health care for both sexes;
- research into effective screening methods for male diseases.

Interestingly, amongst other suggestions, the idea of communicating health messages through popular local male personalities is suggested, and several such men are quoted, in a chapter on 'Men into the Millennium'.

Other health authorities

Local needs assessment drives local action

In 1994, suicide and malignant melanoma (skin cancer) were identified as having higher than average death rates (compared to national ones) in the Dorset population. The recent rise in the suicide mortality rate for men under 44 reflected the national trend. Young men were, therefore, identified as the priority population group for the longer term.

The 1994 Dorset Lifestyle Survey collected data to use to measure future progress towards the then Health of the Nation targets. One key finding was that more than 50% of middle-aged men were overweight (i.e. having a Body Mass Index of over 25).

Deciding on these two local health priorities did not, however, take place as a result of an existing, specific and strategic approach to male health at the population level. They were identified through local health needs assessment and the setting of local priorities within the national policy context of the then government's national health strategy.

Suicide in young men

A health promotion scheme was developed to encourage young men to talk about their problems. A media-led campaign, informed through focus group research, was launched to address the fact that many men preferred trying to solve their problems themselves, as they found it very difficult to talk to someone else about them. The message: 'You've got to be tough to tell someone what's up. Talk about your problems. That way they'll get sorted.' was communicated via local radio announcements, billboard posters and beermats in pubs. There was widespread penetration of the message, including coverage on regional television and other media.

During 1995, development of the campaign was influenced by two unexpected factors: the World Mental Health Day campaign materials proving inappropriate for local use, and a project worker being appointed. Subsequently, a local conference was held on World Mental Health Day to begin to develop a comprehensive local suicide prevention strategy.

Interested professionals attended the event. Local, national and international presentations were made on the relevant issues, for example, on the evidence for effective interventions. Participants were asked to reflect on current practice and identify any gaps.

The following factors helped this recognition and prioritisation in relation to two categories:

(1) male suicide
  - identifying the higher than average rate;
  - the conference and resultant action plan;
(2) male obesity
  - identifying the high numbers of overweight men;
  - the challenge to address the problem.

There were also factors that made it problematic to address male obesity strategically:

- the necessarily complex nature of the response;
- the fact that a similar multi-agency framework to the suicide prevention work did not evolve.

From the strategic point of view, although a suicide policy document was not produced, a detailed multi-agency action was developed using the Ottawa Charter for Health Promotion as a framework. Regarding obesity, a health promotion initiative, the 'Keeping It Up!' campaign was planned and implemented.

By summer 1998, the Suicide Prevention Action Plan had itself led to activity on the ground, including research into the views of young, vulnerable users of local services. *Silent cries*, the report on the Bournemouth area, concluded that young people wanted access to a 24 hour helpline for when crises occurred. It also led to a multi-agency training programme for professionals working with young people. In December 1997, the 'Don't Get Down, Get Help' joint scheme between the youth service, the Samaritans and HealthWorks was launched. The scheme produced 50 000 credit card-style information cards, for distribution to schools and youth clubs over the next three years; all were used in six months, so more were printed.

It is too early to be able to evaluate the direct impact of the schemes that evolved out of the strategic work in Dorset. However, the suicide rate among men under 44 declined in both 1996 and 1997, when the rate fell to its lowest level for many years.

Obstacles and supportive factors

As male health is a newly recognised public health problem it has to compete with other priorities within an already overstretched health care system. Researching material for this chapter helped to identify factors that substantially influenced whether or not a response was likely to develop locally.

Research material for health authority case studies was gathered by questioning relevant staff. Obstacles and supportive factors which were identified as important by health authority staff are given below.

Obstacles

Factors experienced as obstacles, or barriers, to generating a strategic response include:

- the massive agenda of work health authorities have to deal with;
- major reorganisations in the NHS, e.g. health authority mergers, and in other sectors, e.g. local authorities;
- financial pressures, e.g. the need to make efficiency savings;
- competition from other more important local priorities for a health authority;
- the limited capacity of the public health function in some authorities;
- the compartmentalised structure of health promotion units in some authorities;
- a lack of specific strategic direction regarding male health needs within some authorities;
- the dominant, organisational culture and established ways of working.

The last of the above points in the list is an important one, as the institutional obstacles are always the hardest to overcome.

> The barriers and blocks . . . are integral to the ways of working and the culture that predominates in the health service. Innovation, new ways of working, devising strategies to work with men in different settings are not championed. There is a protective preciousness of traditional practice at all levels in . . . the health service which requires radical change. (Johnson, 1997)

Further obstacles identified included the following:

- a resistance to non task-oriented groups, e.g. networks, support and single issue groups;
- a cautious approach to addressing new public health problems, partly due to the emphasis on an evidence base to recommendations for new investment, partly due to the predominance of the medical model and partly due to a perceived level of discomfort and uncertainty in men in key posts considering issues concerning masculinity for themselves;
- the low priority given to male health as part of a public health professional remit: if it is allocated to an individual postholder at all, it is

usually tagged on to his or her remit as a minor responsibility. If the postholder then moves jobs, the male health responsibility is often not reallocated.

Supportive factors

There were, however, factors reported as supportive of strategic development activity at health authority level. These are given below together with a case study that reflects actual experience.

Positive factors include developments in the NHS brought about through *The New NHS* and *Our Healthier Nation* White Papers, e.g. Health Improvement Programmes (HImP), Health Action Zones (HAZ), Healthy Living Centres (HLC), Primary Care Groups and the national performance framework for NHS services.

HImPs, HAZs and HLCs, for example, present good opportunities for a health authority to work in partnership with other local organisations with a public health role. Specifically, the important issue of the health of men in the workplace can be addressed.

The White Paper *Our Healthier Nation*

This policy document had, it was reported, focused attention on several key areas concerning male health, for example:

1. the relevance of life expectancy – and other male health inequalities identifiable within the four national key areas of heart disease and stroke, cancers (especially of the lung, skin and bowel among men), mental health (especially male suicide) and accidents – to the renewed national focus on tackling health inequalities;
2. the opportunity of setting a health inequalities target locally, where there are significant health needs among the male population;
3. the relevance of the three key settings to the health needs of males: a Healthy Workforce and the need to invest in workplace health care and promotion, including the provision of appropriately accessible health advice for men; Healthy Schools and how to make this a reality for boys; and, how to reach and involve males in the community in relation to the Healthy Neighbourhood.

National health campaigns

These were considered in the light of their relevance to local male health issues, such as:

1. the Department of Health's campaign to improve the health of men over 40 in May 1998: a disappointing and lacklustre effort in the end that missed the opportunity to raise the national profile of male health by presenting the problem as a purely social class issue, although it did launch the first ever national leaflet on general health for men;
2. the Europe Against Cancer 1998 theme of 'Men and Cancer' that sought to encourage men to seek help sooner if they thought they might be experiencing signs or symptoms of early cancer.

Topical health issues

These very often attract media and government attention and may often have local relevance, e.g. the impotency drug, Viagra, although, unfortunately, the hype whipped up in this particular case severely damaged its potential to take male health inequality issues forward in a constructive way.

Calderdale and Kirklees Health Authority: a local case study

A brief case study of one health authority serves to illustrate specific examples of successfully using the government's aim to address health inequalities as a leverage opportunity to address male health needs at the local level. The Director of Public Health for Calderdale and Kirklees Health Authority dedicated a whole chapter to the health needs of men and boys in Calderdale and Kirklees in his 1996 report in a deliberate attempt to raise awareness and stimulate a debate locally.

Professor Chris Worth asserts in this report that:

> until recently, the debate has, surprisingly, tended to relate only to disease of the prostate and testicle. (Worth, 1997, p. 12)

He continues:

> Although continuing progress in such sex-specific areas of men's health is to be welcomed, concentrating on these areas ignores the important effects of psycho-social pressures on men within modern society ... men, in so far as they continue to hold positions of power and influence in many areas of social life, can perhaps contribute to the incidence of ill health not only among themselves but also among women (and children). (Worth, 1997, p. 12)

Earlier, he explains:

> I make no apologies for some of the more provocative comments made in the Chapter, but suggest that the approach taken here will allow for a more meaningful debate to be conducted in the district. (Worth, 1997, p. 11)

Health authority annual public health reports have proved a valuable vehicle to highlight issues of specifically male health, for example in Kirklees and Calderdale

- the local suicide rate among males (one of highest nationally) by demonstrating how unemployment and deprivation affect young men in the area;
- the high local rate of orchidopexies, a marker for improved child health, as another small illustration of a male health inequality.

Through presenting specific papers on health inequalities at formal health authority meetings and at several in-house partner agency committees, it has also been possible to successfully raise male health issues, such as the health needs of different localities, heart disease, suicides and other important conditions among males.

Non NHS activity

East Midlands Men's Health Network

Launched in 1989 as a small, informal organisation open to men and women working in the East Pennines area of the NHS Trent Region, the East Midlands Men's Health Network grew to a membership of more than 50 health, education, social and probation service providers from the public and private sectors. Bimonthly meetings, at which male health topics were discussed, peer support was sought and given and information and ideas exchanged at both personal and professional levels, were held up until 1998 when the network changed direction following a review of its activities.

The network – the first of its kind in England – had identified two common problems amongst individuals working with males around health-related needs: feeling isolated and lacking explicit management support. There was a clear and shared recognition that significant unmet need existed amongst males in local communities and that more action was required to respond to it.

Although the network received small amounts of funding from Trent Region, some health authorities in Trent and the Department of Health, as well as small educational grants from drug companies, over the years, it never received recurrent core finance. Fortunately, in the early 1990s, the co-ordination role was taken on by a health promotion specialist at North Derbyshire Health Authority which also then started to provide administrative support for the network.

Despite these difficulties and in the absence of other similar organisations up until 1994, the network took on a national profile as an information source and a point of contact with others working in boys' and men's health throughout the UK. Its major achievements – some of which have been referred to earlier – have included:

- holding the first national men's health conference, 'Men's Health Day', in September 1994 (East Midlands Men's Health Network, 1995);
- establishing the National Men's Health Resource Centre;
- launching the National Men's Health Networking List in 1995 (to be converted into a national database) (East Midlands Men's Health Network, 1997);
- holding a second conference on gender and health and understanding masculinities in December 1995 (East Midlands Men's Health Network, 1996);
- publishing a men's health factsheet and a report for health service purchasers (both funded by the Health Education Authority);
- submitting a response on male health to government during the consultation period for the *Our Healthier Nation* Green Paper.

The East Midlands Men's Health Network, the first national conference and the resource centre have subsequently been cited as good practice in annual reports on the state of the public health in England by the Chief Medical Officer (DOH, 1994; DOH, 1995; DOH, 1996b).

Men's Health Day 1994 contributed to raising the media profile of male health and moving it higher up the agenda within the health sector and the political arena. Both conferences have promoted good practice and provided, along with the networking list, valuable opportunities for workers to get in touch with and support each other. The network as a point of contact, the resource centre and the networking list have been used by a variety of service providers and planners, researchers, trainees and students from health and other areas, public health practitioners, the media and lay people seeking help for health problems. It has often been perceived as 'the only place to go' by different enquirers.

The 1996/7 review identified four important factors to take into account when planning the network's future activities: increased work pressures on co-ordinating group members; the growing difficulty in working across health authority boundaries; the diminished likelihood of securing significant or core funding; and, the establishment of three local networks within the Trent Region (Sheffield, Nottingham and North Derbyshire). The review concluded that the network could no longer continue in the same vein, that it should not duplicate the work of the new local organisations and that it should act as an umbrella structure for the new networks at the regional and national level.

Having completed its first piece of work in this new role – the joint response to the Green Paper from Trent Men's Health Network and workers – the network's remit is to make further joint responses to government on consultative documents concerning health and related issues, e.g. the new strategies on drugs, alcohol, smoking, teenage pregnancy and HIV/AIDS.

Nottingham Men's Health Forum

This forum was launched in October 1995. Its fundamental position is a shared criticism of a biomedical model of men's health and support for a social and cultural one. By adopting a social model of health, the forum acknowledges links between gender, masculinities and health, so that the relative importance, for example, of biogenetic factors compared with psychosocial ones, e.g. growing up as a boy, are recognised when working with men.

The forum's underlying perspectives are that:

- *Various aspects of masculinity probably contribute to many men experiencing poor health*: The socialisation processes involved in the transition from boy to manhood influence men's health-related behaviour, e.g. risk taking, difficulty in expressing feelings, not seeking help (often until being in a crisis). The effects of living in a more privileged position in society often hide much unspoken pain and distress in many men's lives.
- *Traditional gender (as well as class and race) relations* impose rigid polarities that view men as publicly active, strong and dominating and women as decorative, passive, home-making and nurturing. These stereotypes make men (and women) susceptible to illness and need challenging and changing to improve men's health.
- *The forum needs to work at a number of levels* to be effective: awareness raising; multi-agency training for health professionals; and, lobbying for initiatives to be put on the public and political agenda.

The forum has a variety of aims:

- to raise awareness of the physical, psychological and social factors that influence men's health, including gender issues such as masculinity;
- to work with other agencies and organisations to develop strategies to improve men's health;
- to facilitate multi-agency education and training amongst professionals working with men;
- to work alongside minority groups to challenge inequalities in health between the sexes;
- to advocate for male health needs within the policy-making arena.

Members of the forum include statutory and voluntary sector organisations: health and local authorities, including social, probation and education services. There are a broad range of individuals, most with professional backgrounds and including independent lay people.

The forum's general approach is multidimensional: to raise awareness of the probable links between gender, masculinities, power and health; to facilitate networking of health workers to support each other around work with men, and to influence policy at the local level.

Achievements include contributing to the production of Nottingham Health Authority's Public Health Report for 1997/8, for which the theme is the health of men; holding quarterly discussion groups open to the public; holding a high profile seminar series on young men and health; running a city-wide conference; setting up and running a 'Train the Trainers in Masculinity and Health' course for trainers from relevant organisations. The membership is over 70 individuals from a wide range of agencies.

Factors which have helped in building the forum include the members' own experience and resources, e.g. understanding the need for a long-term strategic view and a multifaceted approach and the ability to organise; using positive group dynamics and 1:1 relationships, including the sharing of personal health experiences and concerns that has then led to greater individual emotional engagement in the forum's activities; building good relationships with key health authority staff; the publication of national reports covering men's health over the past few years; the mixed sex membership of the forum.

Hindering factors include the fact that men's health is not a 'trendy' issue; the major organisational change in local health services; the forum's limited resources; the prevailing view that male health is a biological issue, and that 'boys will be boys', which is influenced by the medical model view of the body as a collection of parts; the lack of popular understanding of the probable relationships between masculinities, power and health: in particular, an institutional ignorance of gendered issues, e.g. the blockage among senior management, who pay lip service to the issues and don't actually take on a gender-aware approach in their work.

A change in approach led to taking on a longer term view in the forum's efforts to effect change by deciding to work within the membership's individual and collective energies and limitations and not at the pace of others. This resulted in the forum's activity becoming more effective and sustainable. Future plans include emphasising education and training for service providers and influencing policy-makers.

South Warwickshire Men's Health Network

One of the first on the scene, this network was launched in October 1994. Although it does not make claim to a fundamental position on male health issues, its underlying perspectives are that:

- male health remains a largely unacknowledged issue in its own right and is often subsumed into other health topics, e.g. cancer, without an explicit recognition of different influences on men and women;
- a holistic perspective is important in order to recognise the influence of gender, i.e. sociocultural factors affecting, for example, the way men perceive and deal with their own health and illness.

Members join the network for a variety of reasons. Meeting together to discuss male health and provide support for one another in working with boys and men is a central function of the network.

The membership consists of individuals rather than organisational members. Members have a variety of professional backgrounds including social work, health care and promotion, education, and police.

South Warwickshire Men's Health Network's general approach is to persuade the local health authority to include male health on their agenda. It also organises men-only meetings in order to facilitate networking, discussion, a greater understanding of male health issues, sharing of good practice and the provision of mutual support. It arranges lunchtime seminars on male health issues for representatives and staff from key local health organisations.

This network has already achieved the following.

- Male health was formally addressed at the level of the then Health of the Nation committee within the Department of Public Health at the health authority, following the submission of a discussion paper by a health promotion specialist, but with no really concrete outcome.
- A successful workshop for network members and health authority staff was organised in April 1996 with NHS regional funding.
- Publication of the 'Inquiring into Men's Health' report on South Warwickshire.
- A successful seminar on issues raised by this report for health and other service providers (Broad, 1998).

Factors which have helped in the establishment of this forum include the commitment of members to advocate for the issues and support from South Warwickshire Health Promotion Service, who provide health promotion expertise, administrative support and a small amount of funding.

Factors which have proved a hindrance to the network have included a slow and ambivalent health authority response; network members struggling to attend meetings in work time, as male health is not regarded as a priority by their organisations and, therefore, official permission to do so is not granted; the negative response members often get when attempting to raise issues within their own service area; a possible external and inaccurate perception of the network as a group for gay men or for men coming together for therapeutic activity or counselling.

A change in original approach led to the network becoming more proactive, and this culminated in the health authority agreeing to discuss male health, having initially been reluctant to do so. Themes were allocated for each future network meeting with planned input from a member, e.g. working with young men, men working with men, men and stress. It was also decided to hold meetings both for men only and for men and women in recognition that male health impacted upon both sexes. Many people succeeded in obtaining official permission to attend the workshop in 1996 illustrating a range of different organisations' recognition of the issue.

Future plans of the forum include the following: publishing and marketing the 'Inquiring into Men's Health' report; continuing network meetings and lunchtime seminars; developing a mission statement, aims and objectives; making bids for funds; evaluating the impact of seminars; keeping the health authority informed of progress.

Kirklees Men's Health Network

Launched in December 1995 as part of the Kirklees Health For All Programme, this network stands alone amongst the other local networks in England in its emphasis on lay involvement.

Its key underlying perspectives reflect Health For All principles: community participation and partnership working to enable males to take more control over their health; enabling organisations to be more responsive to male health needs by, for example, involving local men in setting health priorities for the local male population; moving toward a more equitable balance in the attention paid to male and female health issues in society; and addressing the major and multifactorial determinants of poor health.

Members come from the statutory and voluntary sector organisations, local authority, health authority, university, and the local housing association. They are a broad range of individuals: most with professional health-related backgrounds but including lay people. About 25% of the members are women.

The network's general approach has been to research male health needs, to raise awareness of these through local conferences and to network and share relevant information and ideas.

Achievements include two local conferences: Men's Health in October 1996 (Kirklees Men's Health Network, 1996a); and, Improving Men's Health and Well Being in Kirklees in February 1998 (Kirklees Men's Health Network, 1998). Two research reports have been published: Survey of Local Men: The healthiest man and the unhealthiest man you have ever known (Kirklees Men's Health Network, 1996b); and Survey of local health professionals, voluntary sector managers, local politicians and managers of health-related services (Artingstall, 1997).

The 1996 conference, attended by 60 local men, was preceded by a community consultation process, using the Talkback panel, one-to-one interviews and focus groups, in order to identify local men's perceptions of what constitutes a 'healthy' and an 'unhealthy' male. This research was reported back to its participants. The conference identified the following priority areas:

- NHS service provision, including GP and hospital care and screening and health checks;
- young men's health;
- health at work;
- sexual health;
- male health-related attitudes;
- life as you get older.

The 1998 conference involved local males and local organisations meeting together to work out how to respond more effectively to these health and social needs.

There have been other achievements. Male health has been covered in the Calderdale and Kirklees Health Authority Director of Public Health's annual reports for 1996 and 1997. The network has secured funding from the health authority for the local conferences and support in kind from the local authority for 1997/8 and 1998/9. It has been invited to run a male health course by the local adult education centre.

Factors which have helped the network to have an impact are: the commitment of individual members, obtaining financial support, and the championing of male health locally.

Factors which have hindered progress are the disillusionment of members keen to do something due to the time-consuming process of agreeing a shared vision, the lack of formal recognition of the network by local health organisations, insufficient funding for secretarial support, meeting resistance when advocating for some issues, and the difficulty in reaching local males.

A change in approach led to greater emphasis on facilitating communication and better understanding between laymen and professional and voluntary health service providers. This has resulted in the launch of MEN-D, a voluntary organisation of Kirklees men working to improve their health and well being. This was set up in November 1997 to involve more local men. MEN-D – with 20 white and members over 30 years old by the autumn of 1998 – aims to bring local laymen together to discuss health issues and concerns. It recruited by mailshot via the local council and through word of mouth. Two MEN-D representatives attend local men's health network meetings. Problems it encountered were to secure active personal commitment from members and funding, although it initially received a small pump-priming grant from the local council. Its future plans are to develop a group identity, recruit more members and communicate bottom-up with the local network and other important agencies that would benefit from a dialogue with local men.

Kirklees Men's Health Network's future plans include internal restructuring, securing funding for administrative support and making links with the government's new public health agenda in order to translate local dialogue into action on the ground.

In conclusion, as the Director of Public Health commented about the network:

> It recognises the need for an innovative approach which will awaken men's interest in their own good health by involving lay persons and groups in the direction and shape of the debate and its implementation. The Initiative promises a challenging and exciting project relating to understanding men's health and learning about healthy practice. Kirklees Men's Health Network has contributed much to achieving the recommendations on male health made in 1997 by the Calderdale and Kirklees Health Authority. (Worth, 1997, p. 17)

Healthy Norfolk 2000

A second example of local strategic activity within the Health for All framework is Healthy Norfolk 2000 (HN2000). HN2000 is a partnership between organisations that have a responsibility for the health of East Norfolk residents, e.g. the health authority, county and district local authorities and the voluntary sector. A local GP, with an interest in male health as an area he felt had not yet been fully addressed, researched male health policy in part completion of an MSc in Public Health. The report was submitted to HN2000 in August 1995.

In 1994, HN2000 had implemented a campaign to promote testicular self-examination and, the following year, the East Norfolk Health Commission (the health authority), that partly funds HN2000, had recommended that HN2000 extend its activity to encompass other male health needs. The male health policy report was written in response to these local developments and to the Chief Medical Officer's call in 1993 for health authorities to investigate how best to promote boys' and men's health.

The report makes 15 recommendations for local policy directions based on a scientific review of the available evidence, mainly from the UK and North America. Two are general ones and the other thirteen relate to coronary heart disease, alcohol, accidents, violence, and prostate cancer screening. Crucially, the report recommends a gender-sensitive approach, i.e. its aim is:

> not to advocate gender-[sex] specific services for men.... The need is for a gender-sensitive approach, targeting men where they are and appropriately to

their gender.... There is no conflict with the provision of services to women. (Stevenson, 1995, p. 7)

It continues:

Improvements on men's health will come from enabling and encouraging men to take control of their lives rather than from increasing the influence of the medical sphere. (Stevenson, 1995, p. 7)

The Men's Health Forum

The Men's Health Forum was set up in 1994 by the Royal College of Nursing (RCN) in response to a motion at its annual congress. Its original purpose was to implement a parliamentary campaign on male health. As a first step, the RCN commissioned MORI to survey District Directors of Public Health and Chief Administrative Medical Officers throughout the NHS in the UK. This survey, conducted in early 1995, was funded through an educational grant from Merck, Sharp and Dohme, the pharmaceutical company whose products include prostate cancer drugs (MORI, 1995).

Until recently, funding has been one of the forum's perennial problems along with variable and inconsistent support from its founding body, the RCN; the absence of an adequately managed co-ordinator post; inadequate accountability to, and communication with, its membership organisations; and the lack of a strategic vision and clear mission statement. Formally, its vague and woolly aim is to:

provide a platform for interested organisations to discuss, disseminate and promote ideas and information on men's health and the development of good practice. (Men's Health Forum, 1998)

At the time of publication, progress has been made in response to some of these problems. Pfizer, the producer of Viagra, is sponsoring the forum to the tune of £150,000. A membership drive has re-established contact with about 60 membership organisations. A new executive committee has been formed. Finally, further publications are in the pipeline to follow on from its first report, 'The Men's Health Review', produced in 1996, including 'The Public Health Implications of Men's Health' which was launched by Tessa Jowell, Minister for Public Health, at a forum meeting in May 1999.

Unfortunately, since its launch, the forum has too often appeared to speak to one audience only – nursing – and about one issue, in particular – sexual health – as the major male health issue. Major challenges still have to be met: its internal operations must be seen to be more professional; its products must be of a higher quality; its central message must be less ambiguous; and its strategic outlook more considered. The potential of the Men's Health Forum to become a truly independent, broadly represen-

tative national body genuinely interested in male health issues as a public
health problem remains, although it has been seriously damaged.

The Men's Health Trust

Launched in 1997, the trust aims to raise awareness of, provide information
about and promote research into health issues which only affect males. It is
concerned with the lack of public and institutional awareness of male-
specific issues and how this contrasts with progress made with female
health. As Farmer (1998) points out:

> For example, our 1997 survey of South London surgeries found that not one
> had a 'well man' clinic . . . our correspondence . . . tells us that many men find it
> difficult to get information about all male conditions, often because they are too
> embarrassed to see their GP or sometimes even to tell their wives . . . men
> have a particular image or temperament which makes them far less likely than
> a woman to see a doctor about any illness . . . let alone a personal one and
> society goes along with that.

The trust is critical of government policy on screening highlighting, for
example, the lack of action to develop male-specific programmes when
compared with women's cancers.

Such criticisms are inappropriate from two perspectives. Firstly, male-
and female-specific cancers are different in important ways when considering whether or not to screen for them: fundamentally, like is not being
compared with like. Furthermore, there is now government funded
research into cost-effective screening methods for two significant cancers
among males: prostate and bowel cancer. Secondly, advocacy for male-
specific conditions only misses the bigger picture. As the Department of
Health commented on the trust's approach:

> we would like to encourage you to widen your remit to include not only the
> diseases which are specific to men . . . but also those where there is a dis-
> proportionate effect on men's health. (Farmer, 1998)

International case studies

In Germany the issue of male health is very new, has been little discussed
and is not widely understood. Female health has been given more emphasis.

Although not yet publicly recognised, some German national men's
organisations, with pro-feminist and gay-affirmative perspectives, as well as
local groups of more traditional, working class men, are concerned with
broad health issues for males, e.g. gender and masculinity. There has been

some recent media coverage, e.g. the new *Men's Health* magazine (a US import) that targets the straight, fit and rich but doesn't speak to any other type of man.

Dresden Healthy City Project

Historically, the former East Germany has not addressed the health needs of males as a population group at the national level. For the first time since both German reunification and the inception of the Gesundes Dresden project, data on male life expectancy, all- and specific-cause male mortality and health behaviour among males were included in the City Health Profile published in 1997. In response to highlighting these trends, the project is planning a Healthy Workplaces programme to promote the health of men in industry.

Hamburg

The profile of male health in Hamburg began rising in the mid-1990s. The city's AIDS coordinator initiated planning work in early 1996, having become more aware of issues concerning male health through HIV prevention programmes targeting gay and bisexual males and through sex education work with young people. This planning was then actioned by an informal network, there being no official city-wide network or working group on male health. Network members consisted of social scientists, sociologists, social workers, teachers, doctors, psychotherapists and others, some of whom had been very active in male health work for a number of years.

It had become apparent, for example, that there was a need to work in sex-specific and gender-sensitive ways with younger people, as boys and girls have different needs. The AIDS co-ordinator and his co-workers then realised more clearly that there was a significant need for 'boyswork' and for more men to be actively involved in this work in various institutions. These issues were then discussed at several conferences and meetings and covered in both national and regional publications. The availability of general and specific epidemiological data on the health of the male population in Germany, and worldwide, provided sound evidence of the need for such activity.

There were other background developments, too. In the former West Germany, a men's movement had been active at local and regional levels with health sometimes on their agenda. In 1996/7, both a major, national conference, 'Equality – A Challenge for Men', and a European conference, 'Promoting Equality – A Common Issue for Women and Men' had taken place. Neither, however, led to any action on male health issues. It appears that there had only been one major male health conference held in the former West Germany: 'Male Health Means Happiness for Women' organised by the Academy of Health, the Institute for School and Adult Education and the Ecological Foundation in Nordrhein-Westfalen in 1996.

In Hamburg itself, a health promotion conference, 'From Boy to Man – New Ways of Bringing Up Boys' was held in 1995. Little is understood about boys' health in Germany at present, although national studies are underway and smaller scale work is also starting in Hamburg. The conference, therefore, made a significant impact being the first of its kind on boys both in Hamburg and in Germany. About 250 men and women attended.

A new network was then set up for those seeking to take this work forward and a second conference was planned for November 1999. This work was done by the multi-agency Sexuality Working Group of the Hamburg Network of Health Promotion, a network of health organisations, partly financed by the Department of Labour, Health and Social Affairs.

In September 1997, Hamburg held its first men's health conference to bring key individuals and organisations together and begin the process of putting a strategy in place for the city. It was organised by a group of people from non-governmental and governmental organisations.

The conference was held over four stages: two full and two half-day events involving 10 presentations and about 30 workshops. About 150 people – mainly professionals from health, education and social services and a few laymen – were present. Topics covered included male health statistics, boys' and men's health beliefs, researching young men, the male role, male identity, male body image, male sexuality, male mental health, men and sport, and gender-specific resources to handle male life crises. A conference report was published and evaluation was very positive.

Following the conference, the organising group took the work further in several ways. First, they lobbied for a health perspective to be integrated into current regional work on promoting sexual equality for both men and women at different levels in society. Second, they put plans in place to set up a city-, and possibly nationwide, men's health network. Third, they held a meeting in November 1998 on promoting men's health in the workplace to consider issues such as:

- the high incidence of accidents at work and its relationship to male identity issues, e.g. the myth of invulnerability: not using safety equipment, not taking up illness prevention measures etc.;
- the workaholic type of man;
- starting a dialogue between men working in social spheres and those working in economic and industrial areas to examine some of the prejudices and taboos each has about the other;

- what do institutions do to improve opportunities for men (and women) to find a balance between work and career planning and aspects of quality of life, such as partners, families and their own health due to the current economic climate, the fear amongst many men of losing their jobs and how this influences the work they do?;
- how can more men be attracted into social work?

Finally, a proposal and funding bid was put together for a European research and conference project on health and gender in Hamburg for the year 2000.

Vienna

If male health is documented at all in Austria, it is purely at the level of life expectancy. Over the past four years, on the other hand, much work has been done on female health needs: there are now both national and local reports on the health of Austrian females and a number of female health promotion centres have been set up. There are no equivalent male health reports nor any organisations focusing on male health.

The Healthy City Vienna Project has not, until now, directed a special focus at males, although in 1999 it is considering whether or not to introduce certain programmes which target males, e.g. prostate cancer screening, the prevention of injuries and accidents, and suicide. Future health protection programmes may take male-specific behaviour or particular life events into account. Furthermore, elderly men in socially deprived situations faced with homelessness and alcoholism may be prioritised as a special target group (Williamson, 1997a). To this end, the Institute for Social Medicine at the University of Vienna published a report on the health of male citizens in March 1999. It provides data on health problems that relate to the priority areas given above.

The North Western Health Board, Republic of Ireland

Many of the major, national public health problems in the Irish Republic are ones that proportionally affect males more than females, e.g. coronary heart disease, cancer, accidents and HIV/AIDS. Only HIV has so far been addressed specifically as a male health issue at the population level. There has, however, been a growing awareness – including in government at the Department of Health and Children – over recent years that more emphasis is needed on male health needs generally (Williamson, 1997a).

Local developments in the North Western Health Board area (equivalent to a health authority in England) provide an interesting case study, in particular from the perspective of a consultation process that involved local males.

The Board's Health Promotion Service identified the need for a conference on the health of the male population of the counties of Donegal, Leitrim and Sligo for the following reasons:

- local statistics showed significant male health needs, especially in relation to the burden of premature death caused by heart disease, accidents and suicide;
- an evaluation of a schools-based health education programme that found it engaged boys less effectively than it did girls;
- the lack of uptake by fathers of a parent support programme.

The following other background factors contributed to the rationale behind the proposed conference:

- the lack of research-informed knowledge about boys' and men's lives and their health-related attitudes and motivations;
- the gap in availability of appropriate information on male health needs;
- the consequently assumed and confused discussions about boys' and men's lives and how to respond to their health needs;
- a growing realisation that there is a justifiable need to work with males and that what is missing is a clear idea of how to take things forward.

In order to prepare for the conference, a fairly extensive consultation was embarked upon regarding what people felt male social issues and health needs to be, reasons for a conference and what the conference's key themes should be. The process involved three consultation meetings with different groups of local men; a men-only day; and, one consultation meeting with heads of services at the North Western Health Board. Local males were contacted via a mailing to a range of organisations, including health and social care services, the armed services, churches, unions, farmers' organisations, schools and youth clubs. Informal contact was also made by phone with a number of individuals known to be working with males.

The men-only day took place a week before the conference itself and was organised by a group of men from a local community. It was part-funded by the health board and attended by 160 men aged 25–70, who lived in different, and sometimes distant, parts of the region. The venue was designed to be as male-friendly as possible and this was partly created, for example, by an art exhibition on 'Men's Images, Men's Voices'. The day was informal and participative. It involved workshops on issues, such as stress, addictions, male health in general, alternative health care, single fathers, rural men and creating groups. Other features of the day were a monologue about men's issues by a community theatre worker, a film followed by a workshop on fatherhood, demonstrations of the art of sculpting and of pottery, that raised issues to do with participants' perceptions of a disabled man as an artist, and the opportunity to talk with a male doctor (Glenboe Men's Network, 1999).

As a direct result of the men-only day, male health days were organised in three local communities to raise awareness of the issues and encourage local males to make their needs heard. Other proposed developments were the provision of training for men working with males, the setting up of a forum for such men and the development of ways to make contact with younger men.

About 120 people – about the same number of women as men – participated in the actual conference, representing local men from different communities, agencies working with boys and men, the North Western Health Board and the National Department of Health in Dublin. Listening to men talking about their health in the context of their lives was the main theme for day 1. Day 2 revolved around sharing good practice. Again, a male-friendly environment was created in different ways, including displays of artwork by local men and of essays and poems on the subject of 'My Dad is special' by local primary school children.

The chief executive officer of the North Western Health Board opened the conference by stating that he saw it:

> as a means of surfacing and making explicit the issues which affect men's lives, so that the learning could be interpreted and translated into action by the Health Board in its capacity as a planner, policy maker and service provider. (Health Promotion Service, 1999)

He and several senior board management colleagues attended both days and the conference was covered by local and national media. The event led to many board departments reviewing their work in relation to male health, in particular some service providers. It was also subsequently agreed that male health needs be incorporated into the board's wider service plans. One implication of this was that the 1999 Health Promotion Service plan includes the goal of developing more male-friendly primary healthcare services.

Summary

This chapter has reported on progress in one NHS region, and more than ten health authorities where time and finance have been invested to consider male health needs and what action to take about them. However, in the majority of cases, this has not led to any sustained activity either at the strategic level or on the ground. Reported explanations for the largely faltering response include:

- workload and financial pressures;
- the nature and culture of the organisation and the impact of major change on it;
- the perception of male health needs as a low priority.

What appears to have helped progress includes the leverage opportunities offered by:

- the impact of the government's new national health strategy and public health agenda, especially the emphasis on tackling health inequalities;
- relevant national health campaigns;
- relevant topical issues.

Progress by the NHS to address male health needs at the population level has been hard to achieve, shortlived and limited in impact.

Significant activity has been detectable among non-NHS bodies. Some local men's health networks have managed to bring different agencies together. A few have tried to involve local laymen. Some have succeeded in contributing to positive action by the major public health organisations that belong to their local 'health community'. Others have also made an impact nationally. All have helped identify unmet need.

Factors reported by networks to have hindered their efforts at generating a strategic response to male health needs by the local health community include:

- the relative disinterest in and limited understanding of male health as a local issue;
- a lack of funding and of administrative capacity for networks;
- resistance to seeing male health as an important issue;
- inadequate management support of a worker as a network member;
- working in isolation to raise the local profile of male health needs;
- the difficulty in reaching a shared definition of what male health is;
- the challenge of engaging local men.

Factors reported as helping their efforts include:

- local health authority support in various forms;
- the combined resources and experience that members bring to the network;
- a collective commitment, especially to advocacy;
- local and national reports that cover male health needs.

A so-called 'independent, broadly representative, national' forum has been established since 1994; after an unimpressive and shaky start, it has still to fulfil its potential. A handful of single issue male health groups have also been active.

The case studies reported on in this chapter may represent the tip of an iceberg. It is likely, though, that a more accurate image is a collection of chunks of ice bobbing around in close proximity rather than a complete and sizeable single iceberg. These mini-icebergs float and submerge intermittently and information about them rarely gets reported on and disseminated.

It is even more difficult to get a real sense of what might be happening in other European countries, but there are some encouraging examples.

Not only do we not know what is going on up and down the UK, but we may also never be able to learn whether activity has been effective or not, because there is little meaningful evaluation of policy development and of initiatives in place. It, therefore, seems timely, as we approach the eighth anniversary of the official recognition of male health as a national public health problem, to propose that the Department of Health funds a review of progress on addressing male health at the population level since 1993, the date of the Chief Medical Officer's crucial report. This review should be directed by a tightly defined remit to recommend appropriate and effective ways forward at both policy and practice levels.

Further reading

Robertson, S. and Williams, R. (1997) *Men's Health: a handbook for community health professionals*. Community Practitioners' and Health Visitors' Association, London.
A useful short overview of theory and practice intended for the community health practitioner.

Because the majority of material in this chapter is derived from original interviews and internal documents there is very little published on the local efforts, other than a few Annual Public Health Reports. See, for example:

Wilson, S. (1999) *Men's Health. The Annual Report of the Director of Public Health*. Nottingham Health Authority, Nottingham.
and
Worth, C. (1997) *The Director of Public Health's Annual Report 1996*. Calderdale and Kirklees Health Authority, Huddersfield.

Chapter 9
Policy and Progress

In this final chapter we:

- review the reasons why men's health has recently emerged as an issue in public health policy;
- summarise what is known about men's health and make suggestions for research;
- debate whether there should be policies for men's health;
- recommend how research, training, local policy development and service delivery should be gendered so that women and men both benefit;
- and, finally, we describe how the authors intend to take this work forward and suggest how our readers can contribute to progress.

Introduction

This book started from the personal experience of the authors in the health of men, themselves and those they knew well. We hope that some of this motivation has been transmitted to readers and that they will see men's health as an issue that links personal and policy inextricably.

In this chapter our aim is to summarise the material from previous chapters, paying particular attention to the links between the evidence, see Figure 9.1. Part one is concerned with discovering the reasons why men's health has come onto the agenda in social science and in health policy. Much of this material was covered in Chapters 1 and 2. Part two assembles information about the socialisation of men, the resulting diversity of masculinities and the effects on men's health. These were the main themes of Chapters 3 and 4, and the resulting effects on men's health at work were described in Chapters 5 and 6. Part three uses the evidence assembled in Chapters 7 and 8 about health policies at national and local levels, in order to debate how policies for men's health should be developed. In Part four, we recommend how gender, with attention to men's and women's health needs, should be brought into research, training, local policy development, and service delivery and, in particular, how this would impact on the workplace as a key setting.

Men without work

Only the frayed map of a dead language.
Cranes rust in the silted harbour.
All the routes lead to defeat.

The forgotten language of breadwinner
gags in their pursed up mouths.
No work names to prop up lost men.

Now nobody can see them,
fiddling around in sheds. They sense
the vacuum that the end of doing leaves.

They get under their wives' feet.
They push shopping trolleys grudgingly.
Only betting shop and boozer greet
them with the old, rough handshake.

They envy the busy purposes
of younger men who've got to get on.
They find ways of getting through the day.

Canned music receives them now,
aliens in the slippery world of fax and mobile phone
as they slide away, unnoticed,
into the darkest mouth.

(Jackson, 1998)

Finally we explain our own plans for taking this work forward. We suggest that there are diverse ways in which our readers can contribute to the development of men's health.

Men's health 'comes out'

The equity debate

There are the two aspects to the equity debate which relate to health needs and health service provision. For example, in the Health of the Nation strategy (DOH, 1992) there are sections on the health of women, children and older people but not for men. We have shown in Chapter 2 that since the start of accurate epidemiological statistics in the nineteenth century the basic measures of infant mortality and life expectancy show males consistently worse than females. This also applies across industrialised coun-

> It is a paradox that, although men are taken as the norm against which the health needs of women are compared, the needs of men themselves are less visible than the needs of women.

tries. In Britain it is only since the Chief Medical Officer's annual report (DOH, 1993) that attention is being given to male health needs.

Perhaps because of men's reluctance to ask for help, the state has been reluctant to target men's health issues, and so health services are not gendered in the sense of being sensitive to the different needs of males and females. 'Gender and health' has, for the last 20 years, been taken to mean women's health. The recent campaign on depression in men (RCP, 1998) is intended to raise the awareness of male sufferers. But it is also intended to raise the awareness of health workers to look for signs of depression in men who may present with physical signs. Male and female health workers may accept the stereotype that depression is a women's disease.

Past, present and future

In Chapter 2 we have shown the persistence of disadvantage in male infant mortality and life expectancy. Although this information has been publicly available, it did not influence the public health policy debate until 1992 (DOH, 1993). Since then much of the attention has been on the increase in young men's suicide. This is very important, but there is the danger that it avoids examination of the wider and deeper trends.

In Chapter 4 we gave a number of examples of men's health behaviour which is often related to inability to handle emotions in a non-destructive way. Abuse of alcohol and drugs associated with violence are often the coping strategy which damages the individual man's health and also that of women and children he knows.

These behaviours are shown in Chapter 3 to be based in patterns of socialisation of boys and men which are deeply rooted in cultural and social patterns. On the one hand, when we look closely at men's lives we see diversity and this offers hope for positive developments; on the other, there is the persistence of collusion, in many instances supported by the media, in upholding the common masculinity stereotype even if most men don't see themselves fitting it.

How are men to break out of this cycle and to value themselves and others in a world which seems to be giving such strong messages about men having to demonstrate their adverse masculine behaviour? How would you seek to change this in your culture?

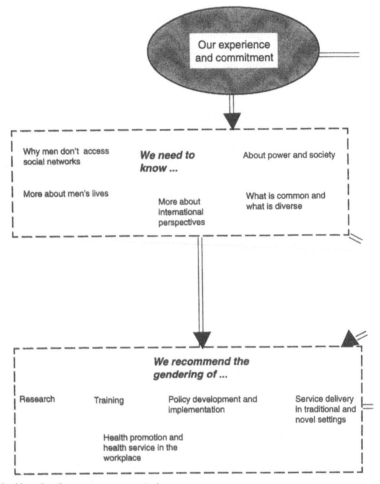

Figure 9.1 How the themes are connected.

Work and unemployment

The effects of work on the health of men have been described in Chapter 5, but the effects of unemployment have not been explored fully. In all age groups males have higher rates of unemployment than females. David Jackson's poem at the beginning of this chapter indicates the impact of the lack of work on older men.

There is a strong link emerging between lack of job security, unemployment and suicide (Lewis and Sloggett, 1998). There may of course be many explanations of this phenomenon, but work does seem to be an issue. The type of 'work' that people do may also be an issue, too much work, not

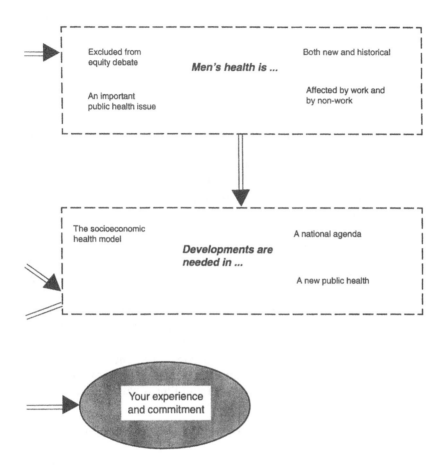

enough work or work of the 'wrong' kind. As Handy (1989) and Sennett (1998) have identified, work can take many forms. For many men it tends to give them their place in society. Often in UK society one of the first questions asked of a man when meeting new people is 'What do you do?' meaning what *work* do you do. It must be hard for some people to say that they have no work, or that they nurse their partner or care for their (or others') children. We have such rigid social expectations, which may be reinforced by media stereotypes. Rethinking what constitutes 'work' and the value of a range of activities to an individual's and a community's health needs to take place.

Think about this issue in relation to a man you know. How would they react to not having paid, traditional work? How did they express their feelings? Did their health suffer? How many men can you remember who did not have a long retirement? Of course, with people retiring earlier this may be changing. An inherent part of work now is insecurity.

A public health issue

Although male health has now been officially recognised as a public health issue in England, its importance, especially relative to female health, and its exact nature require further exploration and a higher profile.

The health of the male population in England and across the industrialised world is characterised by high levels of preventable premature mortality and avoidable ill health. Heart disease and stroke, cancer (of the lung, bowel and skin), accidents and suicide are the major causes of this generalised burden of unnecessary death and illness. However, the major causes vary among different groups of men, according to social class, age, ethnic background and geographical region of residence. Males, as a whole, share similar major preventable health problems, but, within that, different boys and men have diverse health needs.

Males and females suffer both sex-specific ill-health and generic illnesses: the latter, sometimes to the same extent and, at others, to a greater or lesser degree. Not only do boys and men experience health differently to girls and women, but they also interact with health services differently. Research has begun to indicate how males and females differ in their knowledge, attitudes and behaviour in relation to health and illness with gender and the environment.

 What are the implications for the provision of services and for the training of health workers?

What we know and don't know

Men, power and health

It is important to try to understand how power affects men's health. There is the power of the nation state which is particularly evident in the legitimisation of violence in wars leading to death and injury. Acceptance of the power of the state is supported by key social processes such as sport. One of the paradoxes of men's health is that it was the requirement of the state for healthy men to be prepared to kill and be killed which led to the nineteenth century public health developments for children and women.

There is the collective power of the market which defines work and the lack of it and, for example, influences safe practices in the workplace. Then there is the individual power of men over men, over women and over children, which is often expressed through violence or the threat of violence.

The way in which power has been maintained in industrialised countries in the twentieth century largely depends on acceptance of the dominant norms of masculinity.

> It is a paradox that, although few men fit closely the norms in terms of ethnicity, class, physical ability, and sexuality, their attempts to conform and collude with the norms require the suppression of emotions with the harmful effects of drug and alcohol dependence, self-harm in suicide and violence to others.

How acceptable is this concept of male power? Is it a generality of a myth perpetuated by others in society? It is important to remember that some men are equally aggressive to other men and women. How much of this is masculine behaviour or just bad behaviour?

Social networks

Social networks such as 'old boy' networks and men's clubs serve to reinforce the dominance of the mainly male ruling class. Women have shown how these networks together with associated informal practices provide a 'glass ceiling' in organisations which prevents their promotion to senior management. But the majority of men, who do not belong to the dominant class, ethnicity and sexuality, also do not have access to such formal and semiformal social networks.

Women are better than men at creating and maintaining informal social networks. In Chapter 4, in the section Health inequalities and social capital, we argued that the increase in male mortality in Eastern Europe is linked to the isolation of men outside the family and without networks of support. They cannot express their emotional distress to other people and resort to destructive behaviour.

The separation of many men from the positive role of father at the time of the industrial revolution has had harmful effects. It has isolated fathers from a constructive expressive role, and it reinforces for the male child the stereotype of boys and men not having a role in the family other than as the breadwinner.

Diversity and uniformity

There is the danger when describing men's health and discussing the social norms and practices which influence it of assuming uniformity. When we examine health indicators, such as lifestyle factors and measures of mortality, we find wide variations. When we use stratifiers such as class, ethnicity, age, ability, and sexuality, we must remember that each of these covers a range and, when combined, there is a multiplicity of combinations. Connell (1995) has shown in his pioneering empirical research that there are wide variations in masculinities.

There is the paradox that the *apparent* consistency of the dominant norm of masculinity is upheld by such a *diverse* range of men. We use 'apparent' because the norm does change over time and the international comparisons of Hofstede (1998) show differences between countries and cultures.

Are public health planners and health service providers sufficiently aware of this diversity and do they plan and provide services which are responsive to diversity?

Another area where there is the tension between diversity and commonality is in the formation of masculinity in infants and boys. The structure of families varies greatly; the role of the father ranging from absence to full involvement in childcare; much childcare is still provided by women in the family and in nurseries. Yet the dominance of the norms and the consistency of behaviour are strikingly evident.

Research on men's lives

Research into men's lives and the factors which help them maintain good health or influence poor health and illness lags behind that into women's lives (see the Variations in Health research programme (ESRC, 1997)). It is a paradox that, although men are taken as the standard in epidemiology against which women are measured, men are relatively invisible in terms of understanding causal factors compared with women.

In this book we have included extracts from some 'personal stories' of men which do provide understanding of the complexity of influences on men's health throughout their lives. Research of this nature is very limited, however. We need a much wider range of men and much more depth in the stories.

The discussion of fathers has shown the importance of taking a historical perspective, such as from before the industrial revolution, in order to avoid the danger of accepting essentialist arguments about masculinity. Some of the research could be action research, helping fathers to take a more positive role, and arguing for legal constraints and current practice to be more constructive.

Hofstede (1998) has shown that there are wide differences in masculinity and femininity between countries. Further understanding from the international perspective would help to avoid assuming that white Anglo-Saxon culture is the norm.

International perspectives

The study of men's health needs an international perspective for three main reasons: to avoid an 'essentialist' view of the gender socialisation of boys and men and how this affects their health attitudes and behaviour; to learn by comparing the demographic and epidemiological data from different countries; to share ideas and evaluation of policy developments which succeed or fail with respect to men's health.

In Chapter 3 we have described the childhood influences which socialise men, largely with respect to British evidence. There is the danger that we assume this pattern is essential and cannot be changed. But we have some evidence from Australia (Connell, 1995) and the USA (Sabo and Gordon, 1995) which shows diversity within and between nations. Hofstede's (1998) study of over 50 countries has shown that there are differences in national masculinity and femininity with respect to work-related values. This provides striking evidence of differences in gender socialisation.

International comparisons of demographic and epidemiological data, such as those presented in Chapter 2, show some regularities between countries such as male:female birth rate ratios and, in contrast, many variations in the incidence and mortality and morbidity for different conditions. These data provide evidence which needs further exploration in order to build causal models leading to better understanding of social and economic effects on men's health suggested in Figures 9.2 and 9.3 in the next section.

Should there be a national policy?

The socio-economic health model

To understand better the complex interrelationship between factors that contribute to determining the health status of individual males and thus male populations, we adopted the socio-economic model of health suggested by the Independent Inquiry into Inequalities in Health (Acheson, 1998).

The model given in Figure 9.2 illustrates:

the main determinants of health [as] layers of influence, one over another ...
individuals, endowed with age, sex and constitutional factors ... [are sur-
rounded by their] personal behaviour and way of life ... containing factors
such as smoking habits and physical activity ... individuals ... interact with
friends, relatives, and their immediate community, and come under the social
and community influences represented in the next layer. The wider influences
... include their living and working conditions, food supplies and access to
essential goods and services. Overall there are the economic, cultural and
environmental conditions prevalent in society as a whole. (Acheson, 1998,
pp. 5–6)

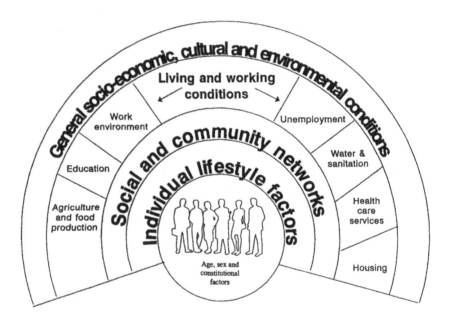

Figure 9.2   The main determinants of health. *Source: Dahlgren & Whitehead, 1991.*

The different influences represented by the five layers interact with each
other over a person's lifetime exposing him or her to various health risks
depending on his or her socio-economic position. As Acheson continues:

These different ... exposures are also important in explaining health
inequalities which exist by ... gender. (Acheson, 1998, p. 6)

The Independent Inquiry's report then gives a second model to show how
the major contributory factors expose different sections of the population
to varying levels of risk to individual health (Figure 9.3). The model is then
used to indicate points where interventions could be made by medical care,

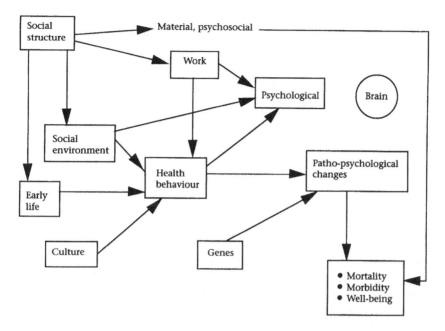

Figure 9.3 Socio-economic circumstances and health outcomes. *Source: International Centre for Health and Society, University College, London, unpublished (1998).*

preventive programmes and public policy. This model could be adapted to illustrate the relationship of gender to socio-economic circumstances – social structure, social environment, work, early life and culture – that influence health status.

In order to promote better male health specifically, this implies broad action on two major fronts: first, research into what are the important contributory factors that cause ill health amongst males and how these factors relate to each other; second, the implementation of a wide range of interventions from the policy arena to focused activity at the very local level. Ways must be found to put initiatives in place that, through meaningful evaluation, will provide evidence of how best to work among boys and men for health gain.

A national agenda

We want to initiate a debate about how best to take things forward five years after the Chief Medical Officer recommended in the mid 1990s that the NHS should investigate ways of promoting male health.

The 1990s saw the national profile of male health raised both as a health issue and a popular issue. Local and national media have given male health concerns more and more coverage and the publishing world has also taken greater interest, as male health has become a newsworthy and marketable topic.

The political and social profile of male health are both starting to take shape, partly due to the health implications of those social issues that affect large numbers of males, such as youth unemployment, labour market trends, crime, violence, school exclusions and educational achievement, being taken more seriously by government. The work of the Social Exclusion Unit has partially acknowledged the gendered nature of social exclusion (SEU, 1997).

Official government recognition of male health as a significant public health problem in 1992 gave a boost to existing activity and stimulated new developments. However, public health and health promotion programmes have tended to evolve sporadically and in a piecemeal way both at the national and local levels – more often than not without adequate evaluation plans in place leading to missed opportunities to find out what effects they had. Fundamentally, there is a lack of a clear sense of where male health sits in the wider public health picture in England.

Despite some small-scale activity initiated by central government, there remains a lack of national direction, co-ordination and leadership to tackle the issue. There is no system in place to register what is happening where, and who is involved. There are no plans as yet at the national level to build a knowledge base of evidence of what works to promote male health and what does not. Despite an initial attempt by the East Midlands Men's Health Network in 1994/5 following the first national men's health conference, there remains no national network for those working with boys and men around their health concerns.

A debate is needed over the next few years to decide what form a national approach to addressing male health needs should take. Simply expecting Health Authorities to find the most effective ways to do so is not a good enough response from government. Options we have considered are:

- a national male health strategy;
- gendering, perhaps 'masculinising', not only existing and future health strategies, but also those in other relevant areas of public policy development, such as 'best value' in local government;
- the introduction of sex-specificity and gender-sensitivity as key themes.

If the government sets a national target concerning health inequalities in its public health strategy, based on 'Our Healthier Nation', specific reference could be made to subtargets in relation to significant sex differences within the whole population.

The NHS could include these themes, for example, when setting standards for the new national performance framework and when issuing guidance to health authorities on service agreements for the commissioning and monitoring of services within the framework of local Health Improvement Programmes.

The expected product of a debate around these and other options would be the formulation of some kind of national framework and, alongside it, a national agenda for research and development into how best to promote male health across society.

A new public health

A public health view shifts the perspective from seeing health problems and their solutions at the level of the individual to a perspective of health needs and concerns at the level of the whole population and, thus, of society. This shift has taken place because although individual responsibility for one's own health was a major theme of the first national health strategy, 'The Health of the Nation' (DOH, 1992), the second strategy, 'Our Healthier Nation' (DOH, 1998a), looks at society at large and recognises public policy as a central tool for improving the population's health.

The 'new public health' reflects these shifts. As Ashton and Seymour (1988) wrote at the time of its emergence:

> the New Public Health is an approach which brings together environmental change and personal preventive measures with appropriate therapeutic interventions.... However, the New Public Health goes beyond an understanding of human biology and recognises the importance of those social aspects of health problems which are caused by lifestyles. In this way it seeks to avoid the trap of blaming the victim. Many contemporary health problems are therefore seen as being social rather than solely individual problems; underlying them are concrete issues of local and national public policy, and what are needed to address these problems are 'Healthy Public Policies' – policies in many fields which support the promotion of health. (Ashton and Seymour, 1988, p. 21)

Male health needs must not be investigated through a telescope trained on the individual boy or man and his body. Significant male health needs (as well as significant female ones) at the population level represent an inequality in health between two sections of the population: boys and men and girls and women. In the same way as the causes of health inequalities can be tracked back into the society itself, so can the chain of factors contributing to the different health needs of the male and the female populations.

The major features of a new public health approach to male health should be:

- a population perspective that allows for the recognition of diverse health needs among different groups of boys and men;
- multidisciplinary mixed method research to better understand male health and how to improve it;
- the Department of Health and the NHS working in partnership across sectors and, in particular, with other agencies that have greater contact with boys and men;
- gendering all public policy and programmes that may have an impact on the health of males;
- consulting with boys and men to ensure health services are accessible to males and responsive to their needs;
- planning interventions based on sound evidence of their effectiveness – and, if no evidence can be found, designing pilot schemes that can be evaluated meaningfully.

Gendering policy and action

Gendering research

In this book we have used our knowledge of a wide range of secondary research together with a much more limited range of primary research to describe what is known about men's health and how the gender socialisation of boys and men affects their health-related attitudes and behaviour. Very little of our evidence comes from research that was designed explicitly to understand these influences. Therefore we make two main proposals.

There is the need for existing research programmes, such as the ESRC (1997) Variations in Health Programme, to pay explicit attention to the influence of gender together with other factors such as class, ethnicity, ability, age, and sexuality.

Much of the research has taken 'gender and health' to mean women's health and, although men have been taken as the norm for comparison, men have remained invisible. It is important that our proposal is not taken to mean that we want to downgrade research on women's health or that men want to take over research being carried out by women. We see the need for some research which is specific by gender and, in particular, for understanding of men's health to catch up with women's. But we believe that women and men will benefit most if the majority of health research recognises gender as a major influence on health attitudes and behaviour and incorporates gender into the research design.

We have provided some personal stories of health-related experiences of men which are extracts from longer life stories.

Our second main proposal is for a wider and more systematic sample of such life stories which will tell us about the interaction of influences and choices in men's lives put into a longitudinal perspective.

However, it has been difficult to get such qualitative research accepted when positivist quantitative research is more acceptable to funders.

Gendering training

With the massive interest and upsurge in women's health and feminist issues, is it surprising that so much energy goes into producing education and training programmes around these issues? Why is men's health not seen as such an interesting and engaging topic for education and training? The data available (see Chapter 2) indicate that men fall behind women in their health status at every stage of their lives.

Perhaps one of the reasons is that a lot of men's health issues seem to be behavioural. There is still a feeling that if a health problem is self-inflicted, either the person themselves feels unable to seek help or the people providing help feel less inclined to assist.

This is a major education area, both of men to modify behaviour to produce less ill health, and of others to reduce the 'blame culture'. For health and social workers' professional training these issues are important. Their future role will be to take the evidence produced by research and best practice and transfer their learning into actions which not only promote the health and social wellbeing of communities, but individuals and groups within those communities. This means that their basic courses of preparation will have to include examples of disparities in health and social wellbeing of those groups. They will also require skills in data analysis, synthesis and discrimination.

As some of the health behaviour of men leads to ill health, those professionals will need to acquire skills and expertise in the behavioural sciences. They will need skills in persuasion, communication, negotiation and promotion. These skills may need to be directed at the general population or at specific groups. These specific groups may be other health and social workers who are not convinced of the need to protect and promote men's health. This suggests a large development programme for education establishments. This is necessary if the health of half the population in the UK is to be served better.

Gendering local policy development

We have identified a strategy and policy vacuum, within which attempts to address male health needs are situated. We have also proposed the development of a new national framework and agenda for male health issues as an umbrella, under which the work necessary to tackle this public health problem can be planned and carried out.

Having rejected the idea of a national male health strategy, we have suggested gendering existing and future public health policy and programmes as our preferred way forward. By this we mean ensuring that policies and programmes, that impact on health inequalities, not only take sex (biological) differences in health into account in a balanced way for males and females, but that they also make due consideration of the influence of gender (sociocultural factors) on health.

Key questions remain, however, such as: where do sex differences sit *vis-à-vis* occupational or social class, ethnic, age and geographical inequalities in health? How can we best address male health needs? What exactly is the Labour government's position on the health (and wider social needs) of boys and men? Some answers may be forthcoming in the much delayed public health White Paper, and second national health strategy for England, *Our Healthier Nation*. At the time of writing, June 1998, this had still not been published.

Progress in England appears to measure up quite promisingly when compared to other European countries. The European Commission has no clear strategic position on male health needs at the level of the European Union population. Although the WHO recently decided not to introduce any gender-specific targets, it has afforded sex differences in health greater recognition having revised its targets for the twenty-first century by introducing gender-specificity as a theme running through the whole of the European Health For All programme. The impact of this policy change remains to be seen. Strategic development activity at the national level is noticeable by its absence in most European countries, with perhaps Switzerland and Germany standing out as having sown some seeds with the potential for germination.

When compared with Australia, for example, things don't look quite as rosy in England, bearing in mind the similarities between the pictures of health among their respective male populations. In 1996, the then Labour federal government drafted the first ever national men's health policy in the industrialised world and several states have men's health policy development in process.

One important difference between the Australian and English experiences to date is that there is as yet no precedent in this country of a national health strategy for a specific population group, whereas this is not the case in Australia. There are, however, important parallels to be drawn between the two situations. National and local government and health services themselves must recognise that many men and many women have different health needs and use health services differently. In order to address these differences among males, models for engaging boys and men in community consultation at the local level need and can be developed.

Evidence of how best to work effectively with boys and men must and can be found, e.g. how to initially reach and involve a specific target group of males in a health intervention. On the one hand, health services will need to reorientate the way they deliver their preventive services to provide them at appropriate points of contact and within appropriate, male-friendly contexts. On the other hand, without more widespread engagement by boys and men in their health issues and a stronger popular and political voice advocating for action, the political will to bring about real change will remain absent.

Advocacy and lobbying are required both at government and health authority levels. Nationally, opportunities for leverage are fairly plentiful at this relatively early stage of the Labour government's term of office. These include:

- the 1995 UK government's commitment to mainstream gender into all policies and programmes;
- the former Chief Medical Officer's (CMO's) call in 1993 to seek ways to promote the health of men;
- The White Papers, *The New NHS* and *Our Healthier Nation*, which include setting national targets, e.g. one on health inequalities, Health Improvement Programmes (HImP) – with local targets, the new national performance framework, Primary Care Groups, Health Action Zones and Healthy Living Centres;
- NHS guidance to health authorities on equity;
- the CMO's project to strengthen the public health function.

The English case studies covered in Chapter 8 illustrated a number of factors that became barriers to developing a strategic approach to male health needs at the local level, including:

- the massive agenda of change overwhelming health authorities including mergers and subsequent reorganisations;
- the dominant organisational culture and established ways of working within some health authorities, that are resistant to peer support networks and single issue groups;
- the lack of readily available and meaningful information on sex differences in health;
- the limited capacity, usually dominated by the medical model, of the health authority public health function;
- male health not being allocated and managed as a major area of responsibility within the remit of public health professionals.

Factors supportive of strategic development to address male health needs include:

- the renewed focus on tackling health inequalities and the ability of health authorities to set a local health inequalities target;
- the official recognition of gender, i.e. sex, as an important paradigm of

health inequalities and the recent increased attention paid to it in research;
- male health being highlighted in national publications;
- male health becoming a more popular and newsworthy issue;
- funding for local men's health networks and a positive working relationship between them and the health authority for their area.

Key points to consider when addressing male health needs at the local level include:

- if setting a health inequalities target for the Health Improvement Programme (HImP), stipulating a subtarget for gender inequalities, if there are significant sex differences locally;
- how to integrate the themes of sex-specificity and gender-sensitivity from male perspectives into existing strategies, policies and programmes;
- the potential benefits of stimulating local debate about the major issues, e.g. through the media;
- how best to enhance social capital and social cohesion amongst local boys and men through 'new public health' programmes;
- working in partnership and taking multifaceted action at different levels to promote male health (from healthier public policy to grassroots community initiatives);
- the relationship between health authority departments, and between organisations within the local 'health community', who share a public health role to promote the health of the male population;
- planning and funding meaningful evaluation of pilot schemes to promote male health in order to be able to report sound evidence of effectiveness;
- being responsive to new evidence from elsewhere of how best to improve boys' and men's health.

Gendering service delivery

Since the late 1970s there has been an interest in women's health. Courses have been offered in 'gender issues' which have focused almost totally on women's health issues. The health of men has, in comparison, not even begun to be addressed. Kimmel (1995) in his introduction as series editor to Sabo and Gordon's (1995) book identifies what he feels is the major problem in raising and sustaining interest in men's health:

> ...masculinity is not only a risk factor in disease etiology but it is also among the most significant barriers to men developing a consciousness about health and illness. 'Real men' don't get sick, and when they do, as we all do, real men

don't complain about it, and they don't seek help until the entire system begins to shut down ... (pp. vii–viii)

If men generally demonstrate lack of interest and concern and do not push for services in their community, who will?

Just as services for women and children have been thought about and developed, services for men need attention. There are attempts in general practice and other community settings to develop services focused on men's health issues. This may be disease specific or 'well men' clinics. There is not, however, a national focus, developments tend to be arbitrary and dependent on local champions. This raises issues about long-term sustainability of these developing services. Both Blaxter (1985) and Bamford (1993) have demonstrated men's poor take up of GP services. Perhaps this is a feature of how services are provided and managed. There needs to be consideration of how men would like to use GP services, do they need male specific sessions? Perhaps just the thought of sitting in a mixed reception area is too much. Can all male clients be guaranteed a male doctor if they require one?

In Chapter 2 there are graphic examples of the morbidity and mortality rates for men which highlight the importance of gendering service delivery for men.

The workplace as a key setting

When looking for a major focus for delivering men's health, the workplace would be an ideal setting. Men who are at work can be identified through employment systems, that is national insurance contributions, tax returns and PAYE. The government, through its consultation paper on the public health (DOH, 1998a), has highlighted 'healthy workplaces' as a focus for activity.

There will be a need to consider how activities will be targeted and focused in workplaces, and how gender-specific issues will be addressed. There are no general health agencies in the public sector who have access to all ranges of workplaces other than the Health and Safety Executive and Local Authority Environmental Health Officers.

It will be important to consider the type of health activity that can take place in the workplace. Initially, it may be important to separate workplace health, i.e. those issues of health associated with the work done from those of a general health nature. This could leave the employer the responsibility of looking after the health of employees, but link into this system general health issues, which could be the responsibility of local health providers.

This may mean that there would need to be some tax incentives for employers to provide occupational health services or subscribe to a locally provided scheme. It could well be that where there is a large employer without an occupational health service, a local Primary Care Group could provide a service as a means of meeting local health needs. This would make workplace health an integral part of primary health care and link employees' health at work into what is already known about their health in general practice.

Whichever approach is taken, the workplace remains an ideal focus for addressing health issues. The major issues to consider include access, defining focus, identifying methods of delivery, a process for monitoring input and for evaluating outcomes.

Final remarks

In this final section the authors set out what we intend to do in order to gain further understanding of men's health and to take the ideas of this book into the local and national policy arena.

Margaret Bamford wants to encourage health professionals to think about men and their health in the same way that they think about women's and children's health. This could be achieved in part by a balanced approach to gender issues being included in all preregistration programmes for the caring professions. This could then be augmented by continuing professional development of individuals. From this preparation would emerge champions, people who would pick up the challenge of addressing men's health in a very broad way. Health care providers can be helped to collect information on local need, targeting services, monitoring and evaluating outcomes and health gain.

Mike Luck feels that writing this book has meant he has been deskbound for over a year. He wants to return to talking with men about their health and writing their stories. He would like to continue working for the development of men's health at the local level with South Warwickshire Men's Health Network and with South Warwickshire Health Promotion Service.

Peter Williamson became a founder member of the planning group formed to set up a men's health institute shortly after completing his contribution to this book. In Spring 1999, the group initiated a consultation process around the establishment of this new institute to be launched in the year 2000. Its principal focus will be the promotion of boys' and men's health with its main activities being advocacy, research into, and development of, effective policy and practice, and the dissemination of evidence-based information. The institute will, for example, take work forward on a number of the key issues highlighted in this chapter as necessary in order to address male health needs more effectively in England during the twenty-first century. Working in partnership with a variety of national and local players, the institute will also build links with like minded agencies in other industrialised countries, including Europe and further afield.

Readers should set their own agendas for action and not forget to reflect on their own personal stories as we have in Chapter 1. This is essential in order to keep strong links between the personal, policy and political perspectives.

In this book we have put emphasis on the workplace as the site for understanding and action. The same needs to be done for schools, neighbourhoods, families. It is up to our readers to take these forward.

References

Acheson, D. (1998) *Independent Inquiry into Inequalities in Health.* The Stationery Office, London.

Ahmad, W. (1993) *'Race' and Health in Contemporary Britain.* Open University Press, Buckingham.

Allsop, J. (1995) *Health Policy and the NHS.* Longman, London.

Anonymous (1979) Health hazards for women working in chemicals and pharmaceuticals, *Industrial Relations Services: Health and Safety Information, Bulletin No. 46* (Oct.), 1–11.

Artingstall, B. (1997) *Survey of Local Health Professionals, Voluntary Sector Managers, Local Politicians and Managers of Health-related Services.* Kirklees Men's Health Network, Huddersfield.

Ashton, J. and Seymour, H. (1988) *The New Public Health.* Oxford University Press, Oxford.

Aveyard, P. (1998) Letter to Peter Williamson, 5th October, from a former Senior Registrar in Public Health, Birmingham Health Authority.

Bamford, M. (1993) Aspects of health among an employed population. Aston University, unpublished PhD Thesis, Birmingham.

Bamford, M. (1996) Public health in the workplace, *British Journal of Community Health Nursing,* **1**, 1, 27–30.

Bamford, M. and Morton-Cooper, A., Dimensions of organisational health, in Morton-Cooper, A. and Bamford, M. (eds.) (1997) *Excellence in Health Care Management.* Blackwell Science, Oxford. pp. 45–74.

Banerjee, A. (1990) Effectiveness of eye protection in the metal working industry, *British Medical Journal,* **301**, 29 Sept., 645–6.

Banks, I. (1997) *Ask Dr Ian about Men's Health.* The Blackstaff Press, Belfast.

Banks, I. and Mason, M. (1998) *Responses to the Green Paper 'Our Healthier Nation' and the Interim Report on Strengthening the Public Health Function.* The Men's Health Forum, London.

Barker, D. (1991) The foetal and infant origins of inequalities in health in Britain, *Journal of Public Health Medicine,* **13**, 2, 64–8.

Barker, D. (1994) *Mothers, Babies, and Disease in Later Life.* BMI, London.

Bentley, M. and Booth, A. (1995) *Putting together a picture of men out bush – strategic directions for rural men's health.* Achieving a Balance – Beyond City Limits Conference. Glenelg, South Australia.

Berrios, G.E. and Shapiro, C.M. (1993) I don't get enough sleep, doctor, *British Medical Journal,* **306**, 843–6.

Birmingham HA (1995) *Closing the Gap. Ten Benchmarks for Equity and Quality in Health.* Birmingham Health Authority, Birmingham.

Blair, A.C.L. (1997) 'The Will to Win' – Speech by the Prime Minister at the Aylesbury Estate, Southwark. Department of Employment, London.

Blaxter, M. (1985) Self-definition of health status and consulting rates in primary care, *The Quarterly Journal of Social Affairs*, **1**, 2, 131–71.

Blaxter, M. (1990) *Health and Lifestyles*. Tavistock, London.

Bond, M. and Williamson, P.R. (1998) *Men's Experiences of Health Problems and Health Services: Summary Report*. North Derbyshire Health Authority, Chesterfield.

Boston Women's Health Collective (1973) *Our Bodies Ourselves*. Simon and Schuster, New York.

Bowlby, J. (1953) *Childcare and the Growth of Love*. Penguin, Harmondsworth.

Bracken, P., Greenslade, L., Griffin, B. and Smyth, M. (1998) Mental health and ethnicity: an Irish dimension, *British Journal of Psychiatry*, **172**, 103–5.

Bradford, N. (1995) *Men's Health Matters. The Complete A–Z of Men's Health*. Vermilion, London.

Brewer, S. (1995) *The Complete Book of Men's Health*. Thorsons, London.

Broad, P. (1998) *Inquiring into men's health – Report on workshop, 12 June*. South Warwickshire Health Promotion Service, Leamington Spa.

Broad, P. and Jenkins, P. (1996) *Developing men's health in Warwickshire. Report of workshop, 23 April*. Warwickshire Health Authority, Warwick.

Broad, P. and Jenkins, P. (1997) *Reference document for purchasers – Gender sensitivity and promoting health*. Warwickshire Health Authority, Warwick.

Brown, C. (1984) *Black and White Britain*. Heinemann, London.

Bruckenwell, P., Jackson, D., Luck, M., Wallace, J. and Watts, J. (1995) *The Crisis in Men's Health*. Community Health UK, Bath.

Bruhn, J.G. and Wolf, S. (1979) *The Roseta Story*. University of Oklahoma Press, Norman.

Bryson, L. (1992) *Welfare and the State*. Macmillan, Basingstoke.

Burgess, A. (1997) *Fatherhood Reclaimed. The making of the modern father*. Vermilion, London.

Burgess, A. and Ruxton, S. (1996) *Men and Their Children. Proposals for public policy*. Institute for Public Policy Research, London.

Busfield, J. (1996) *Men, Women and Madness. Understanding gender and mental disorder*. Macmillan, Basingstoke.

Calnan, M. (1988) The health locus of control: an empirical test, *Health Promotion*, **2**, 4, 323–30.

Carroll, S. (1994) *The Which? Guide to Men's Health*. Consumers Association, London.

Cartwright, A. (1983) *Health Surveys in Practice and Potential*. King Edward's Hospital Fund for London, London.

CEDC (1997) *Alive and Kicking – Final report to the Department of Health*. Coventry Education Development Centre, Coventry.

Christian, H. (1994) *The Making of Anti-sexist Men*. Routledge, London.

Clarke, A. (1998) Stressing the need for dignity at work, *The Times*, Tuesday 25th August, 35.

Clarke, S., Elliott, R. and Osman, J. (1995) Occupational and sickness absence, in F. Drever (ed.) *Occupational Health, Decennial Supplement*. HMSO, London.

Cohen, F. (1986) Paternal contributions to birth defects, *Nursing Clinics of North America*, **21**, 1, 49–64.

Collinson, D. and Hearn, J. (1996) *Men as Managers. Managers as Men.* Sage, London.

Connell, R. (1995) *Masculinities.* Polity Press, Cambridge.

Cooper, M. (1990) *Searching for the Anti-Sexist Man.* Achilles Heel, London.

Cooper, R. (1996) *The Health of Solihull People – The Annual Report of the Director of Public Health.* Solihull Health Authority, Solihull.

Cox, B., Huppert, F. and Whichelow, M. (1993) *The Health and Lifestyle Survey: Seven Years On.* Dartmouth, Aldershot.

CRE (1997) *The Irish in Britain.* Commission For Racial Equality, London.

CSO (1987) *Annual Abstract of Statistics: Industrial Diseases and Fatal Injuries at Work.* HMSO, London.

Currier, C. and Stacey, M. (eds.) (1986) *Concepts of Health, Illness and Disease: A comparative perspective.* Berg Publications, Leamington Spa.

Dahlgren, G. and Whitehead, M. (1991) *Policies and Strategies to Promote Social Equity in Health.* Institute for Futures Studies, Stockholm.

Daniel, W.W. (1968) *Racial Discrimination in Britain.* Penguin, Harmondsworth.

Davey Smith, G., Bartley, M. and Blane, D. (1990) The Black report on socio-economic inequalities in health 10 years on, *British Medical Journal*, **301**, 18–25.

Deakin, M. T. (1998) Letter to Peter Williamson, 8th October, 1998, from the Director of Public Health, Herefordshire Health Authority.

Department of Employment (1972) *Safety and Health at Work* (Robens Report). Cmnd 5034. HMSO, London.

DHSS (1979) *Notes on the Diagnosis of Occupational Disease.* HMSO, London.

DHSS (1988) *On the State of the Public Health for the Year 1987, Annual Report of the CMO of the DHSS.* HMSO, London.

Dobson, M. (1989) Occupational asthma, *Nursing Times*, Nov. 29, **85**(48), 46–8.

DOH (1976) *Prevention and Health: Everybody's Business.* HMSO, London.

DOH (1988) *Report of the Committee of Inquiry into the Future Development of the Public Health Function* (Acheson Report). HMSO, London.

DOH (1992) *The Health of the Nation*, White Paper. HMSO, London.

DOH (1993) *On The State of The Public Health 1992. The Annual Report of the Chief Medical Officer.* HMSO, London.

DOH (1994) *On The State of The Public Health 1993. The Annual Report of the Chief Medical Officer.* HMSO, London.

DOH (1995) *On The State of The Public Health 1994. The Annual Report of the Chief Medical Officer.* HMSO, London.

DOH (1996a) *Variations in Health. What Can The Department of Health and The NHS Do?* Department of Health, London.

DOH (1996b) *On the State of the Public Health 1995. The Annual Report of the Chief Medical Officer.* HMSO, London.

DOH (1997a) *On the State of the Public Health 1997. The Annual Report of the Chief Medical Officer.* HMSO, London.

DOH (1997b) *The New NHS – Modern and Dependable*, White Paper. The Stationery Office, London.

DOH (1998a) *Our Healthier Nation*, Green Paper. The Stationery Office, London.

DOH (1998b) *Chief Medical Officer's Report to Strengthen the Public Health Function – Report of Emerging Findings.* The Stationery Office, London.

Doll, R. (1985) Occupational cancer: A hazard for epidemiologists, *International Journal of Epidemiology*, **14**, 1, 22–31.

Doll, R. and Peto, R. (1981) The causes of cancer, *Journal of the National Cancer Institute*, **66**, 1191–1308.

Doyal, L. (1979) *The Political Economy of Health*. Pluto Press, London.

Doyal, L. (1995) *What Makes Women Sick. Gender and the political economy of health*. Macmillan, Basingstoke.

Drever, F. (ed.) (1995) *Occupational Health, Decennial Supplement. DS 11*. HMSO, London.

Drever, F. and Whitehead, M. (eds.) (1997) *Health Inequalities. Decennial supplement DS 15*. The Stationery Office, London.

Duckworth, D. (1991) Managing psychological trauma in the police service: from the Bradford fire to the Hillsborough crush disaster, *Journal of Social and Occupational Medicine*, **41**, 171–3.

Earwicker, R. (1998) Letter to Peter Williamson, 23rd July. Secretariat of the Independent Inquiry into Inequalities in Health, London.

East Midlands Men's Health Network (1995) *Men's Health Day 1994 – Report of the first national men's health conference*. North Derbyshire Health Authority, Chesterfield.

East Midlands Men's Health Network (1996) *Men's Health Day 1995 – Report of the second national men's health conference*. North Derbyshire Health Authority, Chesterfield.

East Midlands Men's Health Network (1997) *National Men's Health Resource Centre Catalogue* (2nd edn). North Derbyshire Health Authority, Chesterfield.

Edwards, F.C. and McCallum, R.I. (1988) *Fitness for Work*. Oxford Medical Press, Oxford.

Ellicott, S. (1990) Fertile women need not apply, *The Times*, 31 October, 18.

Engel, H.O. and Rycroft, R.J.G. (1988) Dermatology, in F.C. Edwards, R.J. McCallum and P.J. Taylor (eds.) *Fitness for Work*, 114–25. Oxford Medical Publications, Oxford.

Esping-Andersen, G. (1990) *The Three Worlds of Welfare Capitalism*. Polity Press, Cambridge.

ESRC (1997) *Economic and Social Research Council Health Variations Programme Pack*. Lancaster University, Lancaster.

ESRC (1998) *Health Variations Newsletter No. 1*. Lancaster University, Lancaster.

European Commission (1995) *The State of Health in the European Community for 1994*. Commission of the European Communities, Brussels.

Ewles L. and Simnett I. (1992) *Promoting Health: a practical guide*. Scutari, London.

Fagin, L. and Little, M. (1984) *Forsaken Families*. Penguin Books, Harmondsworth.

Farmer, P. (1998) *Submission in response to the Our Healthier Nation Green Paper*. The Men's Health Trust, Bury St Edmunds.

Fletcher, R. (1995) *An Introduction to the New Men's Health*. University of Newcastle, Newcastle.

Furler, L. (1996) Letter announcing the Draft National Men's Health Policy, 30 January, 1996. Australia's Commonwealth Department of Human Services and Health, Canberra.

Gershick, T. and Miller, A. (1995) Coming to terms, in D. Sabo and F. Gordon, *Men's Health and Illness. Gender, Power and the Body*. Sage, Thousand Oaks, CA.

Glasgow Healthy City Project (1994) *Gender and Health – Report of the 1994 Community Conference*. Glasgow Healthy City Project, Glasgow.

Glenboe Men's Network (1999) *Men's Day Out – Report on the day.* Glenboe Men's Network, Bundoran.

Goddard, E. (1991) *Drinking in England and Wales in the late 1980s.* HMSO, London.

Goleman, D. (1995) *Emotional Intelligence.* Bloomsbury, London.

Gott, M. and O'Brien, M. (1990) *The Role of the Nurse in Health Promotion.* Department of Health, London.

Graham, H. (1993) *Hardship and Health in Women's Lives.* Harvester Wheatsheaf, Brighton.

Graham, H. (1998a) Health Variations programme, *Health Variations*, **1**, 2–3.

Graham, H. (1998b) Telephone interview, 1st July, 1998.

Griffin, N. (1992) *Occupational Health Advice As Part Of Primary Health Care.* HSE, London.

Halliday, M. (ed.) (1991) *Our City, Our Health – Ideas for improving health in Sheffield.* Healthy Sheffield 2000, Sheffield.

Ham, C. and Hill, M. (1993) *The Policy Process in the Modern Capitalist State* (2nd edn). Harvester Wheatsheaf, Hemel Hempstead.

Handy, C. (1989) *The Age of Unreason.* Arrow, London.

Hanney, D.R. (1979) *The Symptom Iceberg.* Routledge and Kegan Paul, London.

Harrington, J.M. (1988) Personal communication. University of Birmingham.

Harrington, J.M. and Seaton, A. (1988) A payroll tax for occupational health research, *British Medical Journal*, **296**, 1618.

HAS (1995) *Suicide Prevention. A manual of guidance for purchasers and providers of mental health care.* The NHS Health Advisory Service, Leeds.

Hashemi, K. (1989) *Hazards of the fork lift truck.* MD thesis. University of Birmingham.

Hattersley, L. (1997) Expectation of life by social class, in F. Drever and M. Whitehead (eds.) *Health Inequalities. Decennial supplement DS 15.* The Stationery Office, London.

HDWA (1997) *Men's Health Policy and Discussion Paper.* Health Department of Western Australia, Perth, Australia.

HEA (1991) *The Smoking Epidemic, Counting the Cost to England. West Midlands Region, Volume 12.* Health Education Authority, London.

Health Promotion Service (1999) *Men's Health Conference Report.* North Western Health Board, Ballyshannon.

Hearn, J. (1993) Emotive subjects: Organizational men. Organizational masculinities and the (de)construction of emotions, in S. Fineman (ed.), *Emotions in Organizations.* Sage, London.

Herzlich, C. (1973) *Health and Illness.* Academic Press, London.

Hewlett, B. (1992a) Introduction, in B. Hewlett (ed.), *Father–Child Relations*, Aldine de Gruyter, New York.

Hewlett, B. (1992b) Husband–wife reciprocity and the father–infant relationship among Aka pygmies, in B. Hewlett (ed.), *Father–Child Relations.* Aldine de Gruyter, New York.

Hickman, M. and Walter, B. (1997) *Discrimination and the Irish Community in Britain.* Commission For Racial Equality, London.

Hillis, G. (1998) *6 Monthly Report. January – June 1998.* CPN Department. Birmingham Magistrates Court. Diversion Services, Birmingham.

Hite, S. (1994) *The Hite Report On The Family. Growing up under patriarchy.* Bloomsbury, London.

Hofstede, G. (1980) *Culture's Consequences: International Differences in Work-Related Values.* Sage, Beverly Hills, CA

Hofstede, G. (1981) *Cultures and Organizations: Software of the Mind.* McGraw Hill, London.

Hofstede, G. (1998) *Masculinity and Feminity.* Sage, Thousand Oaks, CA.

Holland, J., Ramazanoglu, C., Sharpe, S. and Thomson, R. (1998) *The Male in the Head.* Tufnell Press, London.

HRSCFCA (1997) *Men's Health – Summary Report. House of Representatives Standing Committee on the Family and Community Affairs.* Parliament of the Commonwealth of Australia, Canberra.

HSC (1998) *Annual Report and Accounts, 1997/98.* Health and Safety Executive, London.

HSE (1981) *First Aid at Work. HS(R)11.* HMSO, London.

HSE (1985) *Health at Work: 1983–85. Employment Medical Advisory Service Report.* HMSO, London.

HSE (1986) *A Guide to the Reporting of Injuries, Diseases, and Dangerous Occurrences Regulations, 1985 (RIDDOR).* HMSO, London.

HSE (1996) *Occupational Dermatitis amongst Jubilee Line Workers. HSE survey results.* Health and Safety Executive, London.

HSE (1998a) *Developing an Occupational Health Strategy for Great Britain. Discussion Document.* Health and Safety Executive, London.

HSE (1998b) *Cutting health risks in the catering and food industry.* Press release. Health and Safety Executive, London.

Hunt, S., McEwen, J. and McKenna, S. (1986) *Measuring Health Status.* Croom Helm, Beckenham.

Hunter, D. (1959) *Health in Industry.* Pelican Books, London.

Hyyppa, M.T. (1991) Promoting good health, *Health Promotion International,* 6, 2, 103–10.

Illich, I. (1976) *Limits to Medicine.* Penguin Books, Harmondsworth.

Jackson, D. (1996) *Breaking Out of the Binary Trap: Boys' Underachievement, Schooling and Gender Relations.* Unpublished.

Jackson, D. (1997) *True Grit in the Men's Ward.* Unpublished.

Jackson, D. (1998) *Screaming Men.* Available from: 13 Mona Rd, Nottingham NG2 5BS.

Jacquinet-Salord, M.C., Kang, T., Fouriaud, C., Nicoulet, I. and Bingham, A. (1993) Sleeping tablet consumption, self-reported quality of sleep, and working conditions, *Journal of Epidemiology and Community Health,* 47, 64–8.

Johnson, A., Wadsworth, J., Wellings, K. and Field, J. with Bradshaw, S. (1994) *Sexual Attitudes and Lifestyles.* Blackwell Scientific Publications, Oxford.

Johnson, M. (1997) *Are they being served? Young men's needs in a school context.* Conference Report. Worcestershire Health Authority, Worcester.

Johnson, M. (1998) Letter to Peter Williamson, 15th October.

Jowell, R., Brook, L., Prior, G. and Taylor, B. (eds.) (1992) *British Social Attitudes: the 9th Report.* Dartmouth, Aldershot.

Kanter, R. (1993) (2nd edn) *Men and Women of the Corporation.* Basic Books, New York.

Kehoe, W. and Katz, R. (1998) Health behaviours and pharmacotherapy, *Annals of Pharmacotherapy*, **32**, 10, 1076–86.

Kenney, J.W. (1992) The consumer's views of health, *Journal of Advanced Nursing*, **17**, 829–34.

Kimmel, M. (1995) Series Editor's Introduction in D. Sabo and F. Gordon (eds.) *Men's Health and Illness. Gender, Power and the Body*. Sage, London.

Kinsey, A., Pomeroy, W. and Martin, C. (1948) *Sexual Behaviour in the Human Male*. W.B. Saunders, Philadelphia.

Kirklees Men's Health Network (1996a) *Men's Health Conference Report*. Kirklees Men's Health Network, Huddersfield.

Kirklees Men's Health Network (1996b) *Survey of Local Men: The healthiest and the unhealthiest man you have ever known*. Kirklees Men's Health Network, Huddersfield.

Kirklees Men's Health Network (1998) *Improving Men's Health and Well-being in Kirklees*. Conference Report. Kirklees Men's Health Network, Huddersfield.

Korda, M. (1997) *Man To Man: Surviving Prostate Cancer*. Little, Brown & Company (UK), London.

Laffrey, S.C. (1986) Development of a health conception scale, *Research in Nursing and Health*, **9**, 2, 107–11.

Le Grand, J. (1982) *The Strategy of Equality*. Allen and Unwin, London.

Lewis, G. and Sloggett, A. (1998) Suicide, deprivation, and unemployment: record linkage study, *British Medical Journal*, **317**, 1283–6.

Lloyd, T. and Wood, T. (eds.) (1996) *What Next For Men?* Working With Men, London.

Long, J. (1991) Let the trained take the strain, *Health Services Journal*, 18th April, 16–17.

Luczynski, Z. (1996) *Issues For Fathers. Paper presented to Nottingham Men's Health Forum*. Personal communication.

Lumb, P. (1998) An early death? Australian men's health policies, in *Proceeding of the Second National Men's Health Conference 1997*. The Men's Health Teaching and Research Unit, Curtin University, Perth.

MacKenzie, B. and Palmer, B. (1996) *Suicide in Young Men. A Prevention Strategy for Dorset*. Conference Report. Dorset Health Commission and Dorset Youth Service.

MacKenzie, B. and Palmer, B. (1997) *Dorset Inter-Agency Suicide Prevention Action Plan*. Dorset Health Commission and Dorset Youth Service.

Marmot, M.G., Shipley, M.J. and Rose, G. (1984) Inequalities in death – specific explanations of a general pattern?, *The Lancet*, May 5, 1003–6.

Marmot, M.G., Davey Smith, G., Stansfield, S., Patel, C., North, F. and Head, J. (1991) Health inequalities amongst British civil servants: the Whitehall II study, *The Lancet*, **337**, June 8, 1387–93.

McClarence, S. (1998) Men of steel try a softer line of work, *The Times*, Saturday 21 November, p. 20.

McCloy, E. (1992) Management of post-incident trauma: a fire service perspective, *Occupational Medicine*, **42**, 163–6.

McDowell, I. and Newell, C. (1987) *Measuring health: A guide to rating scales and questionnaires*. Oxford University Press, Oxford.

McKibbin, R. (1998) *Classes and Cultures. England 1918–1951*. Oxford University Press, Oxford.

Men's Health Forum (1998) *1998 Strategy and Action Plan*. Men's Health Forum, London.

Meth, R. and Pasick, R. (1996) *Men in Therapy*. Guildford Press, New York.

MHPAC (1998) *Strategic Directions in Men's Health – A Discussion Paper*. NSW Health Department, Men's Health Policy Advisory Committee, Sydney.

Modood, T., Berthoud, R., Lakey, J., Nazroo, J., Smith, P., Virdee, S. and Beishon, S. (1997) *Ethnic Minorities in Britain*. Policy Studies Institute, London.

MORI (1995) *Men's health – research study conducted for Reader's Digest*. MORI Social Research, London.

MORI/ICR (1998) *Men's Health. Awareness of Prostate Cancer*. MORI Social Research, London.

Morris, J. (1991) *Pride Against Prejudice*. The Women's Press, London.

Morse, J. and Johnson, J. (1991) *The Illness Experience. Dimensions of Suffering*. Sage, London.

Mustard, J. (1996) Health and social capital, in D. Blane, E. Brunner and R. Wilkinson (eds.) *Health and Social Organization*. Routledge, London.

Nazroo, J.Y. (1997a) *The Health of Britain's Ethnic Minorities*. Policy Studies Institute, London.

Nazroo, J.Y. (1997b) *Ethnicity and Mental Health*. Policy Studies Institute, London.

Nazroo, J.Y. (1998) Ethnicity, in *Health Variations*, **1**, 10–11.

NHSE (1995) *Variations in Health. Report of the Variations Sub-Group of the Chief Medical Officer's Health of the Nation Working Group*. HSG(95)54. National Health Service Executive, Leeds.

NHSE-WM (1994) *Agenda for Health. Report of the Regional Director of Public Health*. NHS Executive West Midlands, Birmingham.

NHSE-WM (1995) *Cancer and Health. Joint Report of the WM Regional DPH and WM Regional Cancer Registry*. NHS Executive West Midlands, Birmingham.

Niven, N. (1989) *Health Psychology*. Churchill Livingstone, London.

Oakley, A. (1972) *Sex, Gender and Society*. Temple Smith, Melbourne.

Oakley, A. (1981) *From Here to Maternity: Becoming a Mother*. Penguin, Harmondsworth.

Oliver, M. (1990) *The Politics of Disablement*. Macmillan, Basingstoke.

Olsen, O. and Kristensen, T.S. (1991) Impact of work environment on cardiovascular diseases in Denmark, *Journal of Epidemiology and Community Health*, **43**, 4–10.

ONS (1995) *The Health of Our Children. Decennial Supplement*. B. Botting (ed.). HMSO, London.

ONS (1997) *The Health of Adult Britain 1841–1994*. J. Charlton and M. Murphy (eds.). The Stationery Office, London.

ONS (1998) *Social Trends 28*. The Stationery Office, London.

OPCS (1992) *General Household Survey*. HMSO, London.

OPCS (1993a) *1991 Census. Report for Great Britain*. HMSO, London.

OPCS (1993b) *1991 Census. Ethnic Group and Country of Birth*. HMSO, London.

OPCS (1994) *1991 Census. Children and Young Adults*. HMSO, London.

Osman, J., Hodgson, J., Hutchings, S., Jones, J., Benn, T. and Elliott, R. (1995) Monitoring occupational disease, in F. Drever (ed.) *Occupational Health, Decennial Supplement. DS 11*. HMSO, London.

Pearse, I. and Crocker, L. (1943) *The Peckham Experiment*. George Allen and Unwin, London.

PHCG (1996) *Draft National Men's Health Policy*. Commonwealth Department of Human Services and Health, Primary Health Care Group, Canberra.

Phillips, A. and Rakusen, J. (1996, revised edition) *The New Our Bodies Ourselves* (British edition). Penguin, Harmondsworth.

Phillips, J. (1984) Rugby, war and the mythology of the New Zealand male, *New Zealand Journal of History*, **18**, 83–103.

Pietila, A. (1994) Factors associated with life control in young men, *Journal of Advanced Nursing*, **20**, 3, 491–9.

Pietila, A. (1998) Life control and health, *International Journal of Circumpolar Health*, **57**, 2–3, 211–17.

Pill, R. and Stott, N.C.H. (1982) Concepts of illness causation and responsibility: Some preliminary data from a sample of working class mothers, *Social Science and Medicine*, **16**, 43–52.

Poulton, E.C. (1978) Blue collar stressors, in C.L. Cooper and R. Payne (eds.) *Stress at Work*. Wiley, Chichester.

Power, C. (1998) Life course influences, *Health Variations*, **1**, 14–15.

Putnam, R. (1993) *Making Democracy Work. Civic Traditions in Modern Italy*. Princeton University Press, Princeton, NJ.

Ramazzini, B. (1713) *Diseases of Workers*. (Translated by W.C. Wright, 1964) Hafner, London.

RCP (1998) *Men Behaving Sadly*. Royal College of Psychiatrists, London.

Reid, M. (1998) Letter from the Director-General, NSW Health Department, launching *Strategic directions in men's health, a discussion paper*, September 1998.

Robertson, S. (1998) Men's health: present practice and future hope, *British Journal of Community Nursing*, **3**, 1, 45–9.

Robertson, S. and Williams, R. (1997) *Men's health: a handbook for community health professionals*. Community Practitioners' & Health Visitors' Association, London.

Rose, J. (1999) Personal communication.

Rotter, J.B. (1954) *Social Learning and Clinical Psychology*. Prentice-Hall, Englewood Cliffs, NJ. (Cited in Niven, N. (1989) *Health Psychology*. London: Churchill Livingstone.)

Royal Commission on Civil Liberties (1987) *Statistics and Costings. Vol. 2*, Cmnd 7054. HMSO, London.

Russell, G. (1983) *The Changing Role of Fathers*. Open University Press, Milton Keynes.

Ryan, J. (ed.) (1995) *Sinews Of The Heart*. Five Leaves, Nottingham.

Rystedt, I. (1985) Work-related eczema in atopics, *Contact Dermatitis*, **12**, 164–71.

Sabo, D. & Gordon, F. (eds.) (1995) *Men's Health and Illness. Gender, Power and the Body*. Sage, London.

Sackville, T. (1995) Under Secretary of State for Health, at the 'Men's Health Matters' Conference, July, London, transcribed from taperecorded proceedings provided by The Medicine Group.

Salisbury J. and Jackson D. (1996) *Challenging Macho Values. Practical ways of working with adolescent boys*. Falmer Press, London.

Sallah, D. (1992) *Assessing the Effectiveness of a Regional Forensic Psychiatric Service*. Aston University, MSc PSM dissertation, Birmingham.

Scrivenor, S. (1991) Gender poser, *The Times*, 28th May.

Segal, L. (1997) *Slow Motion* (update and revised). Virago, London.

Sennett, R. (1998) *The Corrosion of Character: the personal consequences of work in the new capitalism*. W.W. Norton & Co, London.

SEU (1997) *The Social Exclusion Unit*. Cabinet Office Social Exclusion Unit, London.

SEU (1998a) *Truancy and School Exclusion*. Cabinet Office Social Exclusion Unit, London.

SEU (1998b) *Rough Sleeping*. Cabinet Office Social Exclusion Unit, London.

SEU (1998c) *Consultation on Teenage Parenthood*. Cabinet Office Social Exclusion Unit, London.

Silverman, D. (1970) *The Theory of Organisations*. Heinemann, London.

Smith, A. (1992) Setting a strategy for health, *British Medical Journal*, **304**, 457–8.

Smith, A. and Jacobson, B. (eds.) (1988) *The Nation's Health*. King's Fund, London.

Smith, D.J. (1977) *Racial Disadvantage in Britain*. Penguin, Harmondsworth.

Smith, J.A. (1981) The idea of health: a philosophical scale, *Advances in Nursing Science*, **3**, 3, 43–50.

Smith, J. and Harding, S. (1997) Mortality of women and men using alternative social classifications, in *Health Inequalities. Decennial supplement DS 15*, eds. F. Drever and M. Whitehead. The Stationery Office, London.

Smith, S. (1998) Personal communication.

SPPB (1997) *The South Australian Men's Health Background Paper*. South Australian Health Commission, Strategic Policy and Planning Branch, Adelaide.

Stevenson, N. (1995) *Men's Health in Norfolk*. University of East Anglia, Norwich.

Stijkel, A. and van Dijk, F.J.H. (1995) Developments in reproductive risk management, *Occupational and Environmental Medicine*, **52**, pp. 294–303.

Stillion, J. (1995) Premature death in males, in D. Sabo and F. Gordon (eds.) *Men's Health and Illness. Gender, Power and the Body*. Sage, Thousand Oaks.

Taman, A. (1998) Personal communication.

Taylor, G. and Bishop, J. (1991) *Being Deaf: The experience of deafness*. Pinter Publishers, London.

Thackrah, C. (1832) The effects of arts, trades and professions and of civil states and habits on health and longevity, reprinted in Meiklejohn, A. (1957) *The Life and Works of C.T. Thackrah*. E. & S. Livingstone, Edinburgh.

Townsend P. (1979) *Poverty in the UK*. Penguin Books, Harmondsworth.

Townsend, P. and Davidson, N. (1982) *Inequalities in Health*. Penguin, Harmondsworth.

TUC (1988) *Hazards at Work, TUC Guide to Health and Safety*. Trades Union Congress, London.

Tuckett, D. (ed.) (1976) *An Introduction to Medical Sociology*. Tavistock, London.

Valkonen, E. and Pietila, A-M. (1998) Feelings of control and self-assessed health. Work group of European Nurse Researchers, Ninth Biennial Conference, 5–8 July, Helsinki, Finland, in *Knowledge Development: Clinicians and Researchers in Partnership, Proceedings*, Vol. 2.

Waldron, H.A. (1977) Health care of people at work: Exposure to oil mist in industry, *Journal of Social and Occupational Medicine*, **27**, 45–9.

Warren, S. (1996) Who do these boys think they are? an investigation into masculinities in a primary classroom, *International Journal of Inclusive Education*, **1**, 2, 207–22.

Watson, P. (1995) Explaining rising mortality among men in Eastern Europe, *Social Science and Medicine*, **41**, 7, 923–34.

Watson, T. J. (1987) *Sociology, Work and Industry* (2nd edn). Routledge, London.

Watts, J. (1995) *Gendering One. Gendering Two.* Unpublished.

Watts, J. (1997) Personal communication.

Wellings, K., Field, J., Johnson, A. and Wadsworth, J. with Bradshaw, S. (1994) *Sexual Health Behaviour in Britain: the National Survey of Sexual Attitudes and Lifestyles.* Penguin, Harmondsworth.

West, M. (1962) *A Handbook for Occupational Health Nurses.* Edward Arnold, London.

Whitehead, M. (1988) The health divide, reprinted in Townsend, P. and Davidson, N. (1982, revised edition) *Inequalities in Health.* Penguin, Harmondsworth.

WHO (1975) *Environmental and Health Monitoring in Occupational Health.* Technical Report No. 535. World Health Organization, Geneva.

WHO (1985) *Targets For Health For All.* World Health Organization, Copenhagen.

WHO (1986a) *Epidemiology of Occupational Health.* WHO Regional Publication, European Series No. 20. World Health Organization, Copenhagen.

WHO (1986b) *Occupational Health as a Component of Primary Health Care.* World Health Organization, Copenhagen.

WHO (1998a) *Health21 – The Introduction to the Health For All Policy for the WHO European Region*, EUR/RC48/9. WHO Regional Office For Europe, Copenhagen.

WHO (1998b) *Health21 – the Health For All Policy for the WHO European Region – 21 Targets for the 21st Century*, EUR/RC48/10. WHO Regional Office For Europe, Copenhagen.

Wilkinson, H. (1994) *No Turning Back: generations and the genderquake.* Demos, London.

Wilkinson, R. (1996) *Unhealthy Societie*s. Routledge, London.

Wilkinson, R. (1997) Health inequalities: relative or absolute material standards?, *British Medical Journal*, **314**, 591–5.

Williams, F. (1989) *Social Policy. A critical introduction.* Polity Press, Cambridge.

Williams, R. (1983) Concepts of health: An analysis of lay logic, *Sociology*, **17**, 2, 185–205.

Williamson, P.R. (1997a) EU and UK initiatives and policy development in men's health in *Proceedings of the 2nd National Men's Health Conference 1997.* Curtin University, Perth.

Williamson, P.R. (1997b) *One of Us Could Have Been There to Make the Tea, Boyswork – Report on Boyswork Day, Shirebrook School.* North Derbyshire Health Authority, Chesterfield.

Williamson, P. and Jackson, D. (1998) *Joint Response to the 'Our Healthier Nation' Green Paper.* Local men's health networks (East Midlands Men's Health Network, Nottingham Men's Health Forum and Sheffield Men's Health Forum) and men's health workers (North Nottinghamshire) within Trent Region. East Midlands Men's Health Network, Chesterfield.

Wilson, S. (1999) *Men's Health. The Annual Report of the Director of Public Health.* Nottingham Health Authority, Nottingham.

Woodhouse, J. (1998) Letter to Peter Williamson, 25th August, 1998. Director of Public Health, County Durham Health Authority.

Worth, C. (1997) *The Director of Public Health's Annual Report 1996*. Calderdale and Kirklees Health Authority, Huddersfield.

Worth, C. (1998) *The Director of Public Health's Annual Report 1997*. Calderdale and Kirklees Health Authority, Huddersfield.

Wyrobek, A. (1993) Methods and concepts in detecting abnormal reproductive outcomes of paternal origin, *Reproductive Toxicology*, **7** (Supplement 1), 3–16.

Index

Printed and bound by CPI Group (UK) Ltd, Croydon, CR0 4YY

27/10/2024

14580385-0004